[DK] American College of Physicians

HOME MEDICAL GUIDE *to*

DIABETES

D1310186

American College
of Physicians

HOME MEDICAL GUIDE *to*

DIABETES

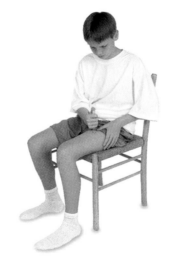

MEDICAL EDITOR
DAVID R. GOLDMANN, MD
ASSOCIATE MEDICAL EDITOR
DAVID A. HOROWITZ, MD

A DORLING KINDERSLEY BOOK

IMPORTANT

The American College of Physicians (ACP) Home Medical Guides provide general information on a wide range of health and medical topics. These books are not substitutes for medical diagnosis, and you should always consult your doctor on personal health matters before undertaking any program of therapy or treatment. Various medical organizations have different guidelines for diagnosis and treatment of the same conditions; the American College of Physicians–American Society of Internal Medicine (ACP–ASIM) has tried to present a reasonable consensus of these opinions.

Material in this book was reviewed by the ACP–ASIM for general medical accuracy and applicability in the United States; however, the information provided herein does not necessarily reflect the specific recommendations or opinions of the ACP–ASIM. The naming of any organization, product, or alternative therapy in these books is not an ACP–ASIM endorsement, and the omission of any such name does not indicate ACP–ASIM disapproval.

DORLING KINDERSLEY
LONDON, NEW YORK, AUCKLAND, DELHI,
JOHANNESBURG, MUNICH, PARIS, AND SYDNEY

DK www.dk.com

Senior Editors Jill Hamilton, Nicki Lampon
Senior Designer Jan English
DTP Design Jason Little
Editor Nick Mulcahy
Medical Consultant David A. Simmons, MD

Senior Managing Editor Martyn Page
Senior Managing Art Editor Bryn Walls

Published in United States in 2000 by
Dorling Kindersley Publishing, Inc.,
95 Madison Avenue, New York, New York 10016

2 4 6 8 10 9 7 5 3 1

Copyright © 2000
Dorling Kindersley Limited, London
Text copyright © 2000 Family Doctor Publications

Based on an original work by Dr. Rudy W. Bilous.

Library of Congress Catalog Card Number 99-76861
ISBN 0-7894-5200-6

Reproduced by Colourscan, Singapore
Printed and bound in the United States by Quebecor World, Taunton, Massachusetts

Contents

INTRODUCTION   *p10*   7

MAKING A DIAGNOSIS   16

TREATING DIABETES WITH DIET   *p21*   19

TREATING DIABETES WITH MEDICATION   29

CHECKING YOUR GLUCOSE LEVELS   40

HYPOGLYCEMIA   *46-53*   46

BREAKING YOUR ROUTINE   *54-55*   54

CHILDREN WITH DIABETES   63

COMPLICATIONS OF DIABETES   *p.75*   *70-72*   *p76-*   68-79

DIABETES CARE   81

FUTURE PROSPECTS FOR DIABETIC PATIENTS   84

QUESTIONS AND ANSWERS   87

USEFUL ADDRESSES   89

NOTES   90

INDEX   *p92*   93

ACKNOWLEDGMENTS   96

Introduction

If you have just found out that you have diabetes, this does not mean that you are sick or an invalid. Millions of people in this country have diabetes, and most lead normal, active lives. Some people with diabetes have had the condition for more than 50 years.

With advances in our understanding of diabetes and improvements in treatment, the prospects for someone with the disease are better than ever. This book should help you understand and control your condition. Doctors now encourage people with diabetes to take considerable responsibility for their own health, pay careful attention to their diet, and perform routine tests on their blood to monitor their progress. You will learn, step by step, how to perform these tests and will develop confidence that you really are in control of your diabetes.

Diabetes is one of the oldest known human diseases. Its full name, diabetes mellitus, comes from the Greek words for siphon and sugar and describes the most obvious symptom of uncontrolled diabetes – the passing of large amounts of urine containing a sugar known as glucose. There are descriptions of the symptoms of diabetes by the ancient Persians, Indians, and Egyptians.

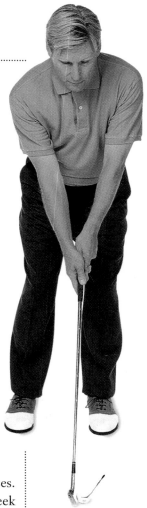

LIVING WITH DIABETES
A diagnosis of diabetes does not mean having to give up everything you enjoy, such as sports. Most people can lead a normal, active life.

However, a thorough understanding of the condition has developed only over the last hundred years or so.

In the latter part of the nineteenth century, two German doctors determined that the pancreas, a large gland behind the stomach, produced some substance that altered the level of blood glucose. In 1921, three Canadian scientists isolated the mystery substance, which they named insulin, from small groups of cells within the pancreas that are called the islets of Langerhans. When insulin became available as a treatment for diabetes after 1922, it was seen as a medical miracle, transforming the future prospects of sufferers and

The Location of the Pancreas

Insulin and glucagon are produced by specialized cells in the pancreas, which also secretes digestive enzymes into the gut. This organ is located behind the stomach.

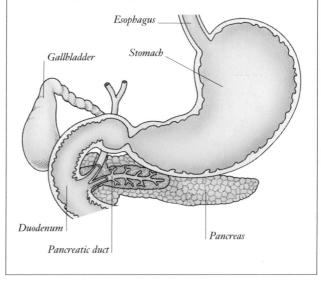

Esophagus

Gallbladder

Stomach

Duodenum

Pancreatic duct

Pancreas

Insulin-producing Cells

This microscope image of cells in the pancreas, magnified 130 times, shows an area of pale pink cells, an insulin-producing islet of Langerhans. This group of cells is surrounded by darker cells that produce digestive enzymes, which are secreted into the gut.

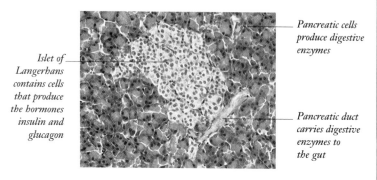

Islet of Langerhans contains cells that produce the hormones insulin and glucagon

Pancreatic cells produce digestive enzymes

Pancreatic duct carries digestive enzymes to the gut

saving the lives of many young people who would otherwise have died after a painful, wasting illness.

About 30 years later, it was discovered that one form of diabetes could be treated with drugs to reduce levels of blood glucose. This new development led doctors to distinguish between two forms of diabetes.

• **Type 1 diabetes** Also called insulin-dependent diabetes mellitus (IDDM), this type most commonly has its onset in younger patients, who need regular injections of insulin to remain healthy.

• **Type 2 diabetes** Also called non-insulin-dependent diabetes mellitus (NIDDM), age-related, or maturity onset diabetes, this form is more common in middle or older age and can usually be controlled by drugs or diet.

WHAT IS DIABETES?

Diabetes is a permanent change in your internal chemistry that results in having too much sugar, or glucose, in your blood. The cause is a deficiency of or resistance to the hormone insulin. A hormone is a chemical messenger that is made in one part of the body, in this case the pancreas, and released into the bloodstream to exert its effect on more distant parts. Complete failure of insulin production results in type 1 diabetes (IDDM). In type 2 diabetes (NIDDM), however, there is usually a combination of a partial failure of insulin production and a reduced body response to the hormone. This is called insulin resistance.

WHAT GOES WRONG?

For several hours after a meal, the glucose in your blood comes from the digestion of food and its processing in the liver. Some glucose is stored, and some is used directly for energy. In the hours after a meal, the body maintains the sugar level in the blood by releasing the stored sugar. After prolonged fasting (overnight or longer), blood sugar is maintained by sugar manufactured in the liver. Insulin is the main hormone responsible for controlling these processes.

Insulin has a unique shape that allows it to plug into special sockets or receptors on the surface of cells throughout the body. By plugging into these receptors, insulin makes cells extract glucose from the blood and prevents them from breaking down proteins and fat. Insulin is the only hormone that reduces blood glucose and it does so in several ways:

Symptoms of Type 1 and Type 2 Diabetes

- Thirst
- Dehydration
- Passing large quantities of urine
- Urinary tract infection or thrush
- Weight loss
- Fatigue and lethargy
- Blurry vision resulting from dehydration of the lenses in the eyes

- By increasing the amount of glucose stored in the liver in the form of glycogen.
- By preventing the liver from releasing too much glucose into the blood.
- By encouraging cells elsewhere in the body to absorb glucose.

Other mechanisms in the body work in conjunction with insulin to help maintain the correct level of blood glucose. However, insulin is the only means the body has of actually lowering blood glucose levels. When the insulin supply fails, the whole system goes out of balance. After a meal, there is no brake on the glucose absorbed from what you have eaten, and the level in your blood keeps rising.

When the glucose concentration exceeds a certain level, the glucose starts to spill out of the bloodstream into the urine. Infections, such as cystitis and thrush, can develop more easily when the urine contains sugar, allowing disease-causing germs to grow more rapidly.

Another consequence of rising blood glucose is a tendency to pass more urine. Extra glucose in the blood is filtered out by the kidneys, which try to dispose of the glucose by excreting more salt and water. This excess urine production is called polyuria, and it is often the earliest sign of diabetes. If nothing is done to halt this process, dehydration and thirst quickly develop. In addition to regulating blood glucose, insulin prevents weight loss and helps build up body tissue. A person whose insulin supply has failed or malfunctioned will inevitably lose some weight.

The severity of these diabetic symptoms and the rate of their development may differ depending on the type of diabetes you have.

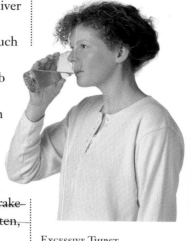

EXCESSIVE THIRST
A person with diabetes will feel perpetually thirsty. This is because an excess amount of fluid is excreted as urine.

TYPE 1 (IDDM)

Since a person with insulin-dependent diabetes mellitus is not producing any insulin, the symptoms can occur very rapidly as control over blood glucose is lost. Insulin has a very important role in maintaining stability in the body by preventing the breakdown of both proteins found in muscle and of fats.

When insulin fails, the by-products of the breakdown of fat and muscle build up in the blood and lead to the production of substances called ketones. If nothing is done to stop this process, the level of ketones will rise until the person develops diabetic ketoacidosis. This is now uncommon because diabetes is usually diagnosed long before the condition develops. However, when diabetic ketoacidosis occurs, patients need urgent hospital treatment with insulin and intravenous fluids.

TYPE 2 (NIDDM)

In people who have type 2, or non-insulin-dependent, diabetes mellitus (NIDDM), the supply of insulin is reduced or it is not quite as effective as normal. Consequently, the blood glucose level rises more slowly after meals than it does in those who are not affected. Since there is less protein and fat breakdown, ketones are produced in much smaller quantities. As a result, the risk of diabetic ketoacidosis is low.

More than three percent of the population in the US are known to have diabetes, and an equal number probably have the disease and are unaware of it. About 90 to 95 percent of diabetics have type 2 diabetes. As the average age and weight of the population increases, type 2 diabetes becomes more prevalent.

WHAT CAUSES IT?

There are several known causes for the reduction of insulin secretion. An individual could be affected by one or more of them.

GENES

Researchers studying identical twins and the family trees of patients with diabetes have found that heredity is an important factor in both kinds of diabetes. With type 1 diabetes (IDDM), there is about a 50 percent chance of one twin developing the condition if the other has it, and a five percent chance of the child of an affected parent doing so. With non-insulin-dependent diabetes, if one of a pair of identical twins develops it, the other will almost certainly do so as well.

Predicting precisely who will inherit the condition is difficult. Certain families have a much stronger tendency to develop diabetes, and scientists have identified several genes that seem to be involved. In these circumstances, it may be possible to test family members and determine their risk of developing the condition.

For the most part, it is not possible to identify the genes involved, unlike a condition such as cystic fibrosis, where a single gene is affected. Even if a close member of your family has diabetes, there is no certainty that you will develop it. Some people who inherit a tendency to diabetes never actually develop the condition. Clearly, other factors are also important.

INFECTION

It has been known for some time that type 1 diabetes in children and young people is more likely to develop at certain times of the year when

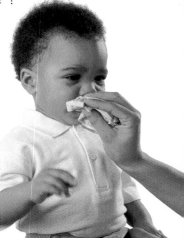

SUSCEPTIBILITY TO DIABETES
Young children tend to develop type 1 diabetes (IDDM) more commonly when they are infected by viruses such as the common cold.

coughs and colds occur. Some viruses, such as mumps and Coxsackie, are known to have the potential to damage the pancreas, causing the onset of diabetes. However, in most patients, it is very rare that doctors can link the onset of diabetes with a specific bout of infection. A possible explanation for this is that the infection may have begun a process that only comes to light many years later.

ENVIRONMENT

People who develop type 2 diabetes are often overweight and have an unbalanced diet. It is interesting to note that people who move from a country with a low risk of diabetes to one with a higher risk have the same chance of developing diabetes as the locals in their new country. Dramatic changes in lifestyle can also increase the likelihood that a person will develop diabetes. The Pacific islanders of Nauru are a good example. These people became very wealthy when phosphates were discovered on their island. Subsequently, their diets changed dramatically. They put on a lot of weight and became much more prone to diabetes.

All of this points to important connections between diet, environment, and diabetes. However, there is no precise link between developing diabetes and the consumption of sugar and sweets.

WEIGHT AND DIABETES
Certain lifestyle factors, such as being overweight, increase the risk of diabetes.

SECONDARY DIABETES

There are a small number of people who develop diabetes as a result of other diseases of the pancreas. For example, pancreatitis, or inflammation of the pancreas, can cause diabetes by destroying large parts of the gland. Diabetes can also be a result of damage to the pancreas caused by chronic alcohol abuse. In some cases, it occurs as a complication of hormonal diseases such as Cushing syndrome, in which the body makes too much steroid hormone, and acromegaly, in which the body makes too much growth hormone. These hormones oppose the effect of insulin on the cells of the body, making it less efficient in metabolizing glucose.

STRESS

Although many people relate the onset of their diabetes to a stressful event such as an accident or other illness, to prove a direct link between stress and diabetes is difficult. The only link may be in the fact that people see their doctors because of some stressful event, and their diabetes is diagnosed at the same time.

KEY POINTS

- Diabetes occurs when an individual cannot make enough insulin, or the insulin that he or she does make is ineffective at controlling blood glucose levels.
- Insulin is a hormone or chemical messenger that is critical for maintaining healthy life.
- Symptoms of diabetes include weight loss, excessive urination, thirst, and lethargy.
- There are several causes of diabetes including genetic factors, infections in the environment, and stress. Any or all of these may be important in an individual case.

Making a diagnosis

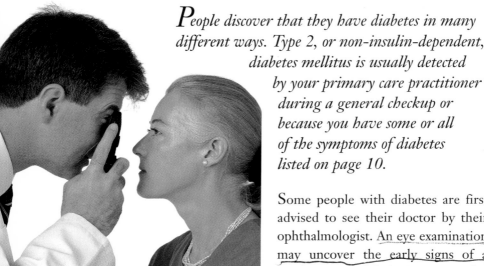

People discover that they have diabetes in many different ways. Type 2, or non-insulin-dependent, diabetes mellitus is usually detected by your primary care practitioner during a general checkup or because you have some or all of the symptoms of diabetes listed on page 10.

Some people with diabetes are first advised to see their doctor by their ophthalmologist. An eye examination may uncover the early signs of a condition called diabetic retinopathy,

VISITING YOUR OPHTHALMOLOGIST
Diabetes is often diagnosed by chance as the result of a visit to the ophthalmologist, who may detect diabetic retinopathy.

changes in the blood vessels of the eye that can develop as a complication of diabetes (see pp.70–72).

If your symptoms suggest that you have diabetes, your doctor will do a blood test to measure your glucose level and ask for a urine sample. The samples may have to be sent to a laboratory for analysis, although many doctors have blood glucose meters in their offices and can give you the results immediately.

Above-average readings from either or both of these tests will probably be sufficient for your doctor to confirm that you have diabetes. Diabetes is commonly treated by your primary care physician rather than a specialist. However, if you or your doctor feel that additional expert opinion is needed, you may be referred to a physician who specializes in diabetes.

As previously mentioned, type 1 diabetes mellitus (IDDM) can have a sudden onset, and the condition may be diagnosed in the hospital at the time of an acute illness such as diabetic ketoacidosis. People with this form of diabetes may continue their care with a specialist. However, many patients with either type 1 or type 2 diabetes receive care from a specialist as well as their primary care physician.

For most patients, the diagnosis is straightforward. In some people, however, glucose levels are borderline or may fluctuate. Under these circumstances, additional testing may be required. These tests may include some or all of the following.

- **High random blood glucose levels** A high level of glucose measured in the blood at any time (above 200 mg/dL) strongly suggests diabetes mellitus.

- **High fasting blood glucose levels** Diabetes mellitus can be confirmed by measuring the level of glucose in the blood after an overnight fast of at least 8 hours. A value of greater than 126 mg/dL on two or more occasions is diagnostic.

- **Oral glucose tolerance test** This test is not usually needed to diagnose diabetes but is more often used to screen for diabetes during pregnancy. After an overnight fast, the patient drinks a specific amount of glucose, and blood levels are measured hourly for several hours thereafter. A level above 200 mg/dL at the two-hour time interval confirms the presence of diabetes.

- **High random glycosylated hemoglobin** The amount of glucose attached to hemoglobin, the oxygen-carrying molecules in the blood, is a good measure of a person's

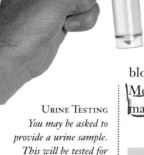

URINE TESTING
You may be asked to provide a urine sample. This will be tested for glucose levels.

average blood glucose level over a two- to three-month period. The test is widely used to monitor glucose control in people who have already been diagnosed with diabetes.

● **Urine tests** Urine can be tested for glucose and ketones. Elevated glucose levels in the urine provide doctors with a clue to diabetes but further blood tests are required to confirm the diagnosis. Measuring ketones in the urine is important in the management of patients with diabetic ketoacidosis.

KEY POINTS

- Diabetes is usually diagnosed from a simple urine or blood test in patients who have symptoms.
- Only a small number of patients need to have more extensive testing.

Treating diabetes with diet

Since there is no cure for diabetes, lifelong treatment is required to control the disorder. The effectiveness of treatment greatly depends on the individual because treatments are generally self-administered. Diabetes can be approached in three main ways: by drugs, insulin, and diet.

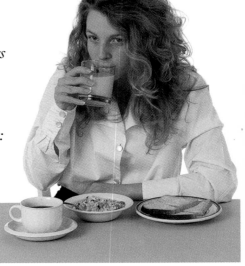

Treating diabetes with diet means following a healthy eating plan rather than a difficult or restrictive diet. This applies to everyone who has diabetes, regardless of the particular type. A healthy diet may be enough to control type 2 diabetes mellitus (NIDDM) in some individuals.

If you have type 1, or insulin-dependent, diabetes mellitus (IDDM), however, you will need to learn how to balance your intake of food with your insulin injections to achieve the best possible control of your blood glucose levels.

Everyone who has type 1 diabetes needs to take insulin by injection, but only a minority of those with

EATING FOR HEALTH
Everyone should follow a healthy diet, but this is particularly important for people with diabetes, since healthy eating helps maintain good glucose levels.

type 2 diabetes are treated this way. For more about insulin, see pages 32–39.

Several different types of drugs are used to control type 2 and will be discussed later (see pp.29–32).

DIET

The diet required for patients with diabetes definitely does not necessitate self-denial. Eat more of the foods that are good for you and cut down on those that are not as good. This is the kind of eating that experts recommend for everyone, not just for people with diabetes. The difference that healthy eating can make in overall health and well-being is even more worthwhile when you have diabetes. Without healthy eating, your medication will not be nearly as effective.

EATING REGULAR MEALS

Your blood glucose is easier to control if you have regular mealtimes. If you are taking insulin, your dietitian or nurse will explain the importance of dovetailing meals with injections. You will gradually develop your own way of matching your food intake to your energy output in order to avoid extreme fluctuations in blood sugar levels.

Matching your food intake and your energy output may be particularly difficult to achieve at first if you are one of those individuals who have unusual working hours, but your diabetic specialist can advise you regarding an appropriate eating schedule. Basically, you should aim to have a substantial meal or a snack every 3–4 hours and work your medication around this schedule. You may need extra meals or snacks when you are working at night.

Example of a Healthy Eating Plan

A well-balanced diet helps control your diabetes and ensures that your medication works effectively. This chart will give you some idea of the foods that you should include in your meals.

BREAKFAST

- Skim or low-fat milk
- Artificial sweetener instead of sugar
- High-fiber cereal, such as oatmeal, branflakes, or shredded wheat
- Wholewheat bread
- Low-sugar jam or marmalade
- Fruit

DINNER

- A starchy food such as bread, potatoes, pasta, rice, or crackers
- At least two portions of vegetables
- Small portions of lean meat or fish; cut off fat and avoid frying
- Fresh or canned fruit in natural, unsweetened juices; with unsweetened/ sugar-free gelatin or custard
- Fat-free or plain yogurt

LUNCH

- Bread, pasta, crackers, or baked potatoes; try low-fat fillings such as lean meat, baked beans, low-fat cheese, or canned fish
- Fresh or canned fruit in natural juice
- Vegetables or salad

SNACKS

- Avoid eating too many snacks if you are trying to lose weight; stick to fruit instead
- Sandwiches or toast with low-fat toppings
- Bowl of cereal or oatmeal
- Low-fat potato chips
- Plain cookies
- Muffins

The Right Weight for Your Height

To find out whether your weight is above or below the normal range for your height, find your current weight on the left side of the chart below. Then run your finger across the chart to your height and see which of the three bands (overweight, a healthy weight, or underweight) you fall into.

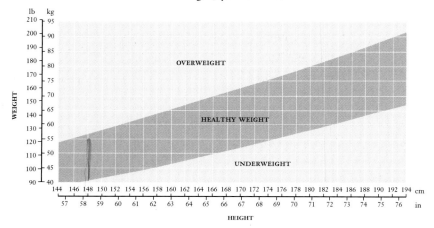

HEIGHT/WEIGHT GRAPH FOR MEN AND WOMEN

CONTROLLING YOUR WEIGHT

People whose diabetes is newly diagnosed may be advised to lose some weight. If you are not sure, check the weight and height chart above.

Once your new eating plan is established, you will probably find that it is easier to maintain a stable weight. In the meantime, it is worth following a few simple guidelines.

Remember that you will lose weight only if you eat less food than your body needs to carry out its daily activities. The information on the following pages can be used as guidelines to healthier eating. There is no reason why everyone in the family should not enjoy the benefits of your "diabetic" diet. However, if some of them are big fans of fried food or desserts, you may find it better to introduce the changes gradually rather than all at once.

Often you will find that you can eat a meal that tastes very much like what you are used to but is better for you because it includes the healthier versions of familiar foods. The healthy eating plan (see p.21) shows how you might do this, substituting the foods listed for your usual ones.

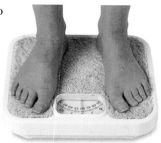

MONITORING WEIGHT
Try to keep to your ideal body weight. Newly diagnosed diabetic patients are often advised to lose some weight.

MAINTAINING A BALANCED DIET

Healthy eating means having a good mix of the right kind of food and cutting back on those that can do more harm than good. If you are confused or worried about what you should eat, see a dietitian for advice. Once you get used to the basics, maintaining a good diet is fairly simple, as shown on the next few pages.

At each meal your food distribution needs to be in the following proportions:

- Two-fifths of your meal should be composed of starchy, high-fiber food.
- Two-fifths of your meal should be composed of vegetables, salad, or fruit.
- The remaining one-fifth of your meal should be a protein source, such as meat, fish, eggs, legumes, or cheese.

All patients should discuss their diet with their nutritionist and physician. For some people it may be important to restrict protein, and in others carbohydrate restriction may

Try These Tips to Lose Weight

- Cut down on fried and fatty foods (see pp.24–25)
- Eat smaller portions
- Cut out snacks such as potato chips and cookies; try fruit instead
- Eat regular meals
- Exercise more

be advised. Fad diets should be avoided. Appropriate diet is essential to achieve and maintain normal weight and desirable blood sugar control.

EATING THE RIGHT CARBOHYDRATES

Carbohydrates are broken down in your body to produce glucose to give you energy. There are two types of carbohydrates: sugars and starches.

● **Sugars** Sugar, candies and chocolate, cakes, cookies and desserts, and sodas are included. You should avoid these foods because the glucose in them gets into your bloodstream very quickly, causing a sudden rise in your blood glucose level. You can use artificial sweeteners, such as saccharine and aspartame, on cereals and in drinks, instead of sugar. It is fine to use a small amount of ordinary sugar for baking cakes, but you should eat these as desserts and do not forget the calorie content!

● **Starches** Bread, potatoes, pasta, rice, cereals, and fruit are good examples. They tend to be absorbed more slowly and release their sugar into the blood more gradually. They are good sources of energy. Eat them regularly and include some with each meal. Individuals vary in their response to different foods. The more you know about your own responses, the better you will be able to manage your diet and control your sugars.

Foods to Avoid
You should avoid sugary carbohydrates in your diet. They will cause a sudden rise in your blood glucose level.

EATING THE RIGHT FATS

The type of fat that we eat is also important. The three main types of fat are saturated, unsaturated, and hydrogenated.

● **Saturated** Saturated or animal fat is found in fatty meats, whole milk, butter, and lard. This type of fat can cause problems for the arteries (see p.76). Everyone needs to reduce the intake of this kind of fat.

● **Unsaturated** These fats are better than saturated fats and come in two forms. Polyunsaturated fats are found in such products as sunflower oil, pure vegetable oil, and corn oil. Monounsaturated fats are found in olive, and safflower oils. This type of fat can be used instead of saturated fat.

● **Hydrogenated** These fats, found in processed foods and margarines, have recently been shown to contribute to elevated cholesterol and circulatory problems and should be avoided.

Remember that all fats are high in calories and could lead to weight gain if consumed in excess.

EATING THE RIGHT FIBER

Fiber, also called roughage, comes from plants. It can be either soluble, which dissolves in water and slows absorption of food, or insoluble, which cannot be digested and helps prevent constipation. Insoluble fiber is also useful when you are dieting because it makes you feel full.

Increasing the fiber content of your diet does not mean having brown rice and bran with everything. However, you should aim to consume about 30 grams of fiber a day. Fiber is essential to keep your intestines working well. Soluble fiber can help with blood glucose control and keeps your blood cholesterol levels down. Foods high in soluble fiber include baked beans, peas, lentil soup, and oatmeal and other oat-based cereals. Foods such as high-fiber cereals, wholewheat bread, pasta, flour, rice, and unpeeled vegetables and fruit contain mainly insoluble fiber.

EATING THE RIGHT PROTEINS —25%

Proteins are necessary so that your body can repair tissue. Proteins also fuel normal growth in children. However, you probably need less than you think. Aim to have about 25 percent of your daily energy requirements in the form of protein.

Protein can come either from cereal sources, such as bread, cereals, rice, pasta, and flour, or from animal sources, such as meat, fish, eggs, and dairy products. Animal proteins tend to be relatively high in fats and calories and contain no carbohydrates. This needs to be taken into account when planning your diet.

AVOIDING SALT

Too much salt is not good for anyone and can lead to high blood pressure. Try to use only a small amount in cooking and do not add more at the table. Herbs, spices, and pepper are better choices to add more flavor to your food.

SUFFICIENT VITAMINS AND MINERALS

If you are eating a well-balanced diet, you do not need vitamin or mineral supplements. Some researchers have suggested that deficiencies of minerals such as chromium and selenium may have a role in the onset of diabetic complications. However, there is no way of measuring either the quantities in your diet or the levels present in your body. It is probably best to eat as varied a diet as possible to ensure that you get enough of these elements along with all other nutrients.

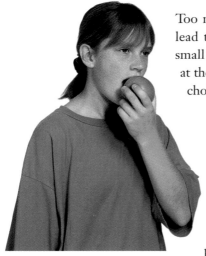

GETTING ENOUGH FIBER
Consume plenty of unpeeled fruit and vegetables, and wholegrain cereals to keep the intestines working well.

Alcohol and Diabetes

Having diabetes does not mean that you cannot drink, but you should follow a few commonsense rules, especially if you are on oral medication or insulin. Remember that alcohol can cause hypoglycemia (see p.47).

- Limit yourself to a moderate amount of alcohol in any one day. Have no more than a single mixed drink, a bottle of beer, or a small glass of wine.
- If you are trying to lose weight, you should remember that alcoholic beverages are high in calories.
- Make sure that you eat a meal containing carbohydrates whenever you drink alcohol.
- Alcoholic beverages may bring on a hypoglycemic attack in people who take medication to control their diabetes.

KEY POINTS

- Eat regularly.
- Include some starchy food or carbohydrate with each meal, choosing high-fiber versions when possible.
- Reduce your fat intake and remember to watch the type of fat that you consume.
- Limit the sugars and sweet foods you eat.
- Aim to keep to your ideal body weight and exercise regularly when possible.
- Use salt sparingly.
- Do not drink too much alcohol.

Treating diabetes with medication

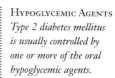

Daily insulin injections are necessary for those individuals who suffer from type 1 diabetes, or insulin-dependent diabetes mellitus (IDDM). People with type 2, or non-insulin-dependent diabetes mellitus (NIDDM), may also find that some form of medication is necessary to control their disorder.

MEDICATION FOR TYPE 2 DIABETES

There are five main kinds of oral medications or pills for people who have been diagnosed with type 2 diabetes mellitus: (1) sulfonylureas, (2) benzoic acid derivatives, (3) biguanides, (4) acarbose, and (5) thiazolidinediones. All of these medications come under the general name of oral hypoglycemic agents (OHAs). They may be taken alone or in combination. Most people with type 2 diabetes find that one or more of these medications, with a healthy eating pattern, keeps their diabetes well under control, although it may take a while to find out which dosage or combination of drugs suits you best. If you experience side effects or find that your blood glucose levels are higher than they should be, go back to your doctor to discuss possible changes to your treatment.

HYPOGLYCEMIC AGENTS
Type 2 diabetes mellitus is usually controlled by one or more of the oral hypoglycemic agents.

Which Sulfonylurea Pills Are Available?

All of these different kinds of sulfonylurea pills stimulate the pancreas to release stored insulin, which raises the level of insulin and thereby helps keep blood glucose levels down.

GENERIC NAME	BRAND NAME	DURATION OF ACTION
Chlorpropamide	Diabinese	Long
Glyburide	Micronase, DiaBeta, Glynase	Medium
Glipizide	Glucotrol, Glucotrol XL	Medium
Glimepiride	Amaryl	Medium

SULFONYLUREAS (SUs)

Sulfonylureas, commonly known as SUs, work by stimulating the pancreas to release stored insulin and thereby help keep down blood glucose. You have to remember that, although you are not actually taking insulin, these pills have a similar effect because they increase the amount of insulin in your bloodstream. It is possible for insulin to increase too much. If this happens, your blood glucose levels will drop too far, and you may sometimes experience the symptoms of hypoglycemia (see p.47). To prevent this from happening, make sure that you eat regularly and take your pills either with or just before a meal.

As with insulin, the duration of action of SUs varies (see chart above) and they must be taken once, twice, or three times a day depending on how fast they work. The long-acting preparations may not be best for older people or those whose lifestyle makes it difficult to have regular meals because of the risk of hypoglycemia.

Apart from the risk of low blood glucose, most people taking SUs have few if any serious side effects. Probably the most annoying side effect is that your face can get very flushed and hot when drinking alcohol. The precise reasons for this reaction are unclear. SUs lower your blood glucose and make you feel very hungry. You could gain a lot of weight if you are not careful. A minority of people are not able to take SUs because they are allergic to them.

BENZOIC ACID DERIVATIVES

Repaglinide is a new drug marketed under the brand name Prandin. Although it works by the same mechanism as the sulfonylureas, chemically it is a benzoic acid derivative, rather than an SU. It is very short-acting and is designed to be taken before each meal to decrease the rise in blood sugar that follows the meal.

BIGUANIDES

Only one biguanide, metformin, is available in the US. No one is sure precisely how metformin works, but it increases the effects of insulin on the liver. Your blood glucose level will not drop too far when you are on metformin because it does not stimulate the release of insulin. The drug is often prescribed for people who are overweight because it does not make you feel hungry or gain weight. You normally start on a low dose, taking it once or twice a day with meals, and then gradually build up the amount taken. Metformin must be avoided in patients with kidney complications (see pp.72–73). The main side effects of metformin are nausea and diarrhea, which may be troublesome enough to cause some people to stop taking this medication.

ACARBOSE

This drug works by interfering with the breakdown of carbohydrates into sugar, thereby increasing absorption of glucose from food. Unfortunately, this means that more sugars remain unabsorbed in the large intestine where many bacteria and microorganisms live. These feed on the abundant sugar and proliferate, which can result in loose stools and gas.

THIAZOLIDINEDIONES

This newer class of drugs improves the body's sensitivity to insulin and thus enables the hormone to lower blood glucose more effectively. The first drug in this group, troglitazone, has been shown to be very effective, but users have been warned by the Food and Drug Administration that their liver function should be monitored monthly for the first year. This drug is no longer used as first-line therapy. A second type of thiazolidinedione, rosiglitazone, has recently been released under the brand name Avandia.

MEDICATION FOR TYPE 1 DIABETES

When you have type 1, or insulin-dependent diabetes, there is no alternative to replacing the missing insulin by means of daily injections. Some people with type 2, or non-insulin-dependent, diabetes may not adequately control their blood sugar with diet and pills and must change to a regimen of insulin injections. If you have recently had to make this change, you may need time to adjust to the idea. However, with the right information and support from your diabetes care team, you will soon be able to control your diabetes effectively. Your health-care professionals will show you how to give injections and manage your condition. Do not worry if you need to see your diabetes specialists several times to make things clear. In fact, they will encourage you to keep asking questions and coming back until you feel com-fortable with the mass of new information. We will now consider some of the questions people with newly diagnosed diabetes ask most often.

WHY INJECT THE INSULIN?

Injecting insulin is the only effective way of getting it into your bloodstream. If you swallow insulin, it is partly digested and becomes less active and therefore cannot do its job of controlling your blood glucose level. Although other ways of giving insulin have been tried, they all have problems. Injection is the only practical option available at this time.

WHY INJECT UNDER THE SKIN?

In theory, insulin could be injected into a vein or a muscle. In practice, however, injecting the insulin into a vein several times a day would be difficult, and intra-muscular injections can be painful. Both of these methods are sometimes used in special circumstances, especially when you are ill or cannot eat regularly.

WHAT TYPES OF INSULIN ARE THERE?

Insulins can be divided into short-, medium-, and long-acting varieties. The short-acting insulins are always clear. Currently available preparation types include

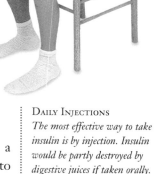

DAILY INJECTIONS
The most effective way to take insulin is by injection. Insulin would be partly destroyed by digestive juices if taken orally.

Regular (R), Semilente, and Humalog (lispro). Longer-acting preparations are cloudy because of the buffers added to slow down their absorption from the skin. Medium-acting preparations include NPH (N) and Lente (L). The main long-acting preparation currently available is Ultralente (UL). Short-acting insulins are frequently mixed in the same syringe with other longer-acting insulins. Since it is important not to contaminate clear insulin with cloudy insulin, you should always draw up the clear preparation into the syringe first.

In the past, insulin was prepared from animal sources, mainly beef and pork. In the last two decades, these insulins have been predominantly replaced by genetically engineered human insulin. The last available preparations of animal insulin will soon be removed from the market. If you are still using animal insulin, you should consult your doctor.

Do not confuse the type of insulin with the manufacturer. Iletin, Humulin, and Novolin are simply brand names. It is the R, N, UL, or Humalog that will tell you the type of insulin regardless of the brand.

WHY INJECT SEVERAL TIMES A DAY?

The object of insulin therapy is to imitate the body's behavior as closely as possible. In a person who does not have diabetes, insulin is released by the pancreas in response to food (see diagram opposite). As the blood glucose level falls between meals, the insulin level drops back toward zero. However, the insulin level never quite reaches zero. There is no time in the 24 hours when there is no detectable insulin in the bloodstream. With insulin injections, you are trying to reproduce the normal pattern of insulin production from the pancreas.

Levels of Insulin and Blood Glucose

These graphs of the levels of glucose and insulin in the blood show the normal pattern of insulin release and the way in which insulin injections relate to mealtimes.

KEY:

NATURALLY RELEASED INSULIN

SHORT-ACTING INSULIN

MEDIUM-ACTING INSULIN

BLOOD GLUCOSE

NORMAL PATTERN OF INSULIN RELEASE

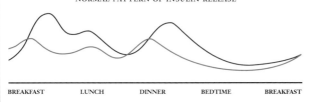

BREAKFAST   LUNCH   DINNER   BEDTIME   BREAKFAST

NATURAL INSULIN RELEASE
In a person who does not have diabetes, insulin is released by the pancreas in response to the rise in blood glucose levels produced by eating food.

INSULIN RELEASE WITH MULTIPLE INJECTIONS

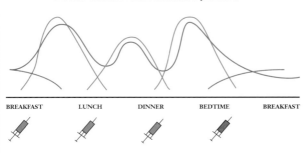

BREAKFAST   LUNCH   DINNER   BEDTIME   BREAKFAST

BEFORE MEALS PLUS NIGHT
To reproduce normal conditions, many people inject themselves with short-acting insulin three times a day before meals, plus a nighttime injection of medium- or long-acting insulin to control blood glucose overnight. Mealtimes are flexible with this method.

INSULIN RELEASE WITH TWICE DAILY INJECTIONS

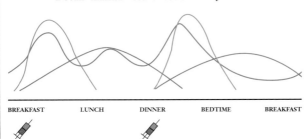

BREAKFAST   LUNCH   DINNER   BEDTIME   BREAKFAST

TWO TYPES TWICE DAILY
Two injections a day of both short- and medium-acting insulins cover the meal you are about to have as well as a later meal or overnight. Meal timing is important to avoid low glucose levels.

There are several ways of injecting insulin, using different types of insulin and numbers of injections per day. For example, many people follow a system of three injections of short-acting insulin before the three main meals of the day, plus a nighttime injection of a medium- or long-acting insulin to control blood glucose during sleep. Other methods involve two injections a day of a mixture of short- and medium-acting insulins. The short-acting component covers the meal you are about to have, such as breakfast or dinner, while the medium-acting component covers you at lunch or overnight. The regimen you use will depend on the type of diabetes you have, your response to different insulins, and the personal preferences of you and your doctor.

If you cannot or do not want to give yourself several injections a day, or have only a partial deficit of insulin, you may be able to use just one or two daily injections of medium- or long-acting insulin.

HOW AND WHERE DO I INJECT MYSELF?

Your diabetes care team will show you how to do the injections and explain the various types of equipment available. Many people today use disposable plastic syringes and needles, although some still prefer the glass ones with disposable needles. Disposable syringes and needles can be used many times with little risk of infection. They are usually thrown away when injections are less comfortable because the needle is blunt.

Insulin injection pens are also very popular, largely because of their convenience and portability. There are several types of pens to choose from, but the principles governing their use are much the same. Consequently, it is simply a matter of which one suits you best.

Insulin Injection Sites

The thighs, abdomen, upper arms, and buttocks are the main sites at which to inject insulin. Most people learn how to inject themselves in just a few days.

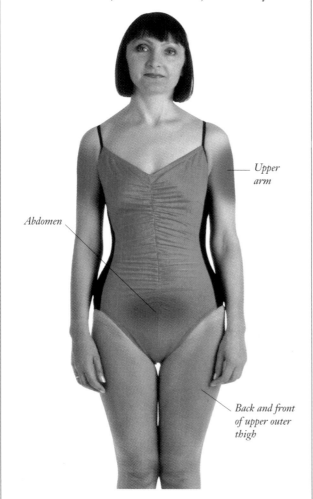

Upper arm

Abdomen

Back and front of upper outer thigh

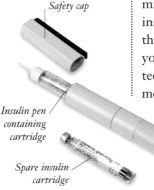

Safety cap

Insulin pen containing cartridge

Spare insulin cartridge

INSULIN PENS
Many people prefer to use insulin pens rather than the more traditional syringes and needles. Insulin pens are simple to use and can be carried around easily.

Recent research has suggested that some people may mistakenly insert the needle at the wrong depth so that insulin goes into the muscle beneath the skin. Judging the depth accurately can be quite difficult, especially if you are slim. However, it is important to master the technique because insulin can be absorbed from muscle more rapidly than from under the skin.

Your diabetes care team will show you how to inject insulin correctly. A lot of people find that the simplest way is to pinch the skin and inject the bunched up area at an angle of 90 degrees. Do not pinch the skin too hard because it will hurt when the needle goes in.

Patients who have difficulty with inadvertent muscular injection should discuss this problem with their diabetes specialist. There are different lengths of needle available to help with injections.

You will be given advice about the best sites for injection (see p.37). The tops of the thighs, buttocks, abdomen, and upper arms are the most common sites; it is best to avoid using the same area every time because you could develop a small fatty lump, called lipohyper-trophy, that could affect insulin absorption.

External insulin pumps provide an alternative to injections. Insulin is delivered to the body through a tube with a needle inserted under the skin, and a refillable cartridge holds insulin for two days. The pump is set to give a steady trickle under the skin throughout the day.

WILL THE INJECTIONS HURT OR LEAVE MARKS?

People who have been giving themselves injections for years say they do not feel a thing, but many beginners may experience slight pain at first. Try to be as relaxed as possible and follow the technique you have been shown. Some people find it helps to rub and numb their skin with ice for a few seconds before the injection. You might try this technique.

With practice, you should find that the injections rarely hurt. However, if things do not improve, ask your doctor or nurse specialist for advice about the problem.

The needles are very fine and usually do not leave a mark. Sometimes you may get a little bleeding or even a bruise after an injection, but this is nothing to worry about. You have probably punctured one of the tiny blood vessels under the skin, which happens from time to time. There is virtually no chance of insulin directly entering the bloodstream.

KEY POINTS

- Drug treatment is useful for patients with type 2 diabetes (NIDDM).
- Drugs work in different ways and have different side effects. Talk to your doctor about your prescription.
- Insulin injections are necessary for all type 1 and a significant percentage of type 2 diabetes patients.
- Usually at least two and as many as four injections may be needed a day.
- Insulin preparations can be short-, medium-, or long-acting.
- Premixed short- and medium-acting preparations are available.
- Injections rarely cause discomfort or leave a mark.

Checking your glucose levels

The goal of all treatment for diabetes, whether it is diet, drugs, or insulin, is to keep the levels of glucose in your bloodstream as near to normal as possible. The closer you get to achieving this, the better you will feel, especially in the long term.

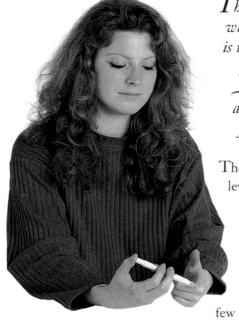

SELF-TESTING
The special device that is being used here allows you to take a drop of blood for testing and monitoring your blood glucose levels.

There are two methods to monitor glucose levels yourself: blood tests and urine tests. Your doctor or nurse will advise you about which one to use, and how often to do the checks. Neither test is difficult once you become accustomed to it.

The development of simple finger-prick blood testing methods in the last few years has transformed life for patients taking insulin. Close monitoring of glucose levels is very useful when you are on insulin because it allows you to make adjustments to your dose depending on the results.

When your diabetes is controlled by drugs and/or your diet, urine tests can give you nearly as much information as blood tests. Urine tests may also be much more convenient, although they are not commonly used.

There are also blood tests that measure an average blood glucose level over an extended period before the test, which may be from two to eight weeks. We will look at each of these three approaches.

Meter reading

BLOOD TESTS

Systems are available for self-blood-glucose monitoring, or SBGM. They give accurate results and help you improve blood glucose control. They are also useful if you suspect you may be about to have a hypoglycemic reaction (see pp.46–53). Taking an exact reading will either reassure you that all is well or confirm that you need to take action.

The tests are done on a drop of blood from your fingertip. The glucose in the drop of your blood reacts with a pad or pads on the end of a plastic strip. The strip is then inserted into the appropriate meter, which gives a reading. There are many different meters and strips available, each of which has a different reaction time. Consequently, it is vital to follow the manufacturer's instructions carefully.

Testing strip

BLOOD TESTING
Special meters are available to read your blood testing strips. The strip, dabbed with a drop of blood, is placed in the meter, which then gives a very precise reading.

HOW TO DO THE TEST

The main drawback of blood tests is that they require a finger-prick sample of your own blood. Of course, someone else may occasionally be able to do this for you. Pricking your finger can be problematic if you are a manual worker or have very sensitive fingers. Rather than having to stab yourself, you might find it easier to use one of the devices that incorporates a spring-loaded lancet. This device also allows you to adjust the depth of the prick.

URINE TESTS

Glucose appears in your urine when your kidneys can no longer reabsorb the amount being filtered from the bloodstream. The problem with urine testing is that this "overflow point" is not the same for everyone. The medical term for this overflow point is the kidney, or renal, threshold. Some people who do not have diabetes have a low threshold. They often need a blood test to confirm this fact and to help determine why glucose has appeared in their urine.

The normal kidney threshold occurs when the blood glucose level is about 180 milligrams per deciliter (mg/dL). For a person with diabetes, a negative urine test can mean that the blood glucose level is likely to be less than 180 mg/dL depending on the personal threshold. A positive test, on the other hand, does not tell you the exact level of blood glucose or by how much it exceeds your own personal threshold.

Despite this relative lack of accuracy, testing your urine and getting mostly negative results may be all you need to confirm that your diabetes is well controlled, especially if you are being treated with drugs and/or you are following a healthy diet. Urine testing, however, is no longer routinely used to monitor control of diabetes.

HOW TO DO THE URINE TEST

Most people use stick tests similar to those used for testing blood glucose. You dip a stick either into the stream of urine or into a specimen you have just passed, then wait for the chemical reaction that results in a color change. Then read the color against

Color chart

Strip for testing urine

TESTING YOUR URINE
A urine test cannot tell you the exact level of your blood glucose, but only if the level is too high.

the chart, which is usually printed on the side of the container. As with the blood testing sticks, how long you wait varies from one type of urine stick to another. Always check the manufacturer's instructions. The test must be done on fresh urine to reflect the level of glucose in your blood at the time of the test. You should empty your bladder about half an hour before the test. Pass another sample about half an hour later and check that fresh sample.

WHAT THE RESULTS SHOW

When you do a blood test, you are really measuring how effective your previous dose of insulin or medication has been. In other words, doing a test just before lunch will tell you the effect of your early morning injection of quick-acting insulin. In the same way, if you do the test before breakfast, it will reflect the effectiveness of the previous nighttime dose.

If you are using insulin, testing frequently and consistently will allow you and your doctor to adjust your insulin doses carefully to achieve optimal control. The most common pattern of testing is before each meal and at bedtime. Sometimes, tests after meals or during the night will be required. Testing is also critical for the detection, treatment, and prevention of hypoglycemia (see pp.46–53). Discuss with your doctor or health-care professional a program for regularly testing, reporting, and evaluating the results.

People on oral medications will also benefit from testing. The relationship between the results of a given test and the specific dose of medication is usually not as direct as for insulin and will vary based on the type of medication used. The pattern of testing will therefore vary. Since blood sugar levels vary throughout the day, a representative sample is helpful to establish any patterns in your daily fluctuations. Patients on insulin or pills should keep a written log of their results and bring it with them on each visit to their diabetes care center.

LABORATORY MONITORING

If you have insulin-dependent diabetes, there will be situations in which your medical advisors will want to assess the effectiveness of your treatment by means of more sophisticated blood tests. These tests are not a substitute for your own routine testing but can provide additional information to help the doctor decide whether your treatment needs adjustment.

GLYCOSYLATED HEMOGLOBIN

This test measures your average blood glucose level over a period of 6–8 weeks. However, as with all averages, your average blood glucose level could be the result of lots of small variations or much larger swings in either direction. For this reason, the glycosylated hemoglobin test is not useful for making day-to-day adjustments of insulin treatment but is a good guide to determine whether your treatment is working well overall. Hemoglobin A_{1C} is the standard glycosylated hemoglobin test now routinely used by physicians to follow the patient's condition and should be performed regularly.

SPECIAL BLOOD TESTING
Periodically, a larger blood sample may be taken to perform an average blood glucose estimate.

KEY POINTS

- Blood tests provide more accurate information about glucose control than do urine tests.
- Blood tests are also more helpful in excluding hypoglycemia or low blood glucose.
- Urine tests are adequate for monitoring patients on diet control or low doses of oral hypoglycemic agents but are not very helpful for alerting patients to hypoglycemia or for making more precise adjustments in medication dosage.

Hypoglycemia

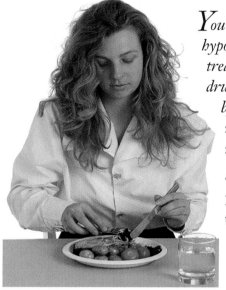

You need to be concerned about hypoglycemia only if you are being treated with insulin or sulfonylurea drugs. If your diabetes is controlled by diet, or if you are taking metformin or acarbose, you will not experience this problem.

EATING AT THE RIGHT TIME
Regular mealtimes, and meals that include carbohydrates, will help ensure that you keep your blood glucose levels under control. Eating every 3–4 hours is sensible.

"Hypoglycemia" means low blood glucose. In a person who does not have diabetes, the levels of blood glucose rarely fall below 60 mg/dL because the natural control system will sense the drop and correct the situation by stopping insulin secretion and releasing other hormones, such as glucagon, which boost blood glucose. In addition, the person will feel hungry, eat, and the blood glucose level will increase as a result.

When you are taking insulin or sulfonylureas, this feedback system no longer operates. Once you have taken insulin or stimulated its production with drugs, you cannot switch it off again. Your blood glucose will continue to drop until you eat some carbohydrates. As the blood glucose level falls, it usually triggers a variety of warning symptoms (see opposite). Hypoglycemia is dangerous because the brain is almost entirely dependent on glucose for normal functioning.

If levels drop too low, the brain works less well and the symptoms shown in the box develop. If the level drops even lower, unconsciousness or coma may result.

PREVENTING HYPOGLYCEMIA

In the past, someone who was starting on insulin might have had to go through a deliberately induced hypoglycemic reaction so that he or she would know how it felt. These days your doctor is unlikely to suggest this because it is not very pleasant. Doing a blood glucose test at home allows you to find out quickly and easily whether your level is getting too low and take action if necessary.

Symptoms of Hypoglycemia

You should be aware of the symptoms of hypoglycemia so that you can take appropriate action. Frequent hypoglycemic attacks may indicate that your treatment or eating pattern needs adjusting.

Sometimes, people suffering from low blood glucose may behave oddly, and others may suspect that they are drunk. Most people who take insulin can use their symptoms as a signal to eat some food. However, symptoms and their severity vary according to the individual. Some people feel hungry before noticing anything else, while others experience tingling around the lips or shakiness. You may not experience all of the symptoms listed below, but it is common to have a headache after suffering a hypoglycemic attack.

- Feeling sweaty or cold and clammy
- Trembling and feeling weak
- Tingling around the lips
- Feeling hungry
- Blurry vision

- Feeling irritable, upset, or angry
- Unable to concentrate
- Looking pale
- Feeling drowsy and losing consciousness if nothing is done

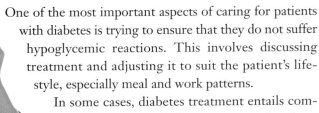

AN IMPENDING
HYPOGLYCEMIC ATTACK
*It is important to recognize
initial symptoms. These can
include feeling sweaty or
clammy, blurry vision,
and drowsiness.*

One of the most important aspects of caring for patients with diabetes is trying to ensure that they do not suffer hypoglycemic reactions. This involves discussing treatment and adjusting it to suit the patient's lifestyle, especially meal and work patterns.

In some cases, diabetes treatment entails compromises. You usually have to accept that there is no alternative but to stick to regular mealtimes, no matter how inconvenient. However, with the wide range of different insulins and injection devices, it is usually possible to arrive at a treatment program that will suit you.

Having regular hypoglycemic attacks is a sign that you need to go back to your doctor or nurse to see how your treatment and/or your eating patterns can be adjusted to prevent the attacks.

WHAT CAUSES ATTACKS?

You will soon recognize the situations in which you are especially vulnerable, but the most common are:

• Eating later than you had planned, which is bound to happen sometimes. If you have had your insulin injection and then miss a meal, eat a small carbohydrate snack.

• A burst of unexpected physical exertion (for more on exercise, see pp.54–55).

• An illness, if it affects your appetite.

• Making an error in either the timing or the dose of your medication.

• Drinking too much alcohol. Your liver cannot produce glucose when it has to break down excessive quantities of alcohol. You will be told not to drink too much alcohol if you are on insulin or are taking sulfonylureas. In addition, you should eat something whenever you drink alcohol.

Having a Hypoglycemic Attack

In hypoglycemia, a low level of glucose in the blood deprives brain cells of their energy source. This condition can occur in diabetes sufferers who are on insulin or sulfonylurea medication.

POSSIBLE CAUSES

- A delayed or missed meal or snack
- More exercise than usual, including things such as gardening, strenuous housework, or sports
- An illness that causes you to eat less than usual
- Medication errors
- Excessive alcohol consumption

TREATMENT

- Consume a quick-acting carbohydrate, such as hard candies or orange juice.
- Afterward, eat some slower-acting carbohydrate such as a sandwich or toast.
- Check your blood glucose level if possible.
- Take more glucose if your symptoms persist.
- If you are due to have a meal or snack, eat something immediately.
- If your symptoms persist, seek medical advice.

TREATING AN ATTACK

A hypoglycemic reaction that is relatively mild can usually be treated with a high-energy drink or orange juice. Remember, diet drinks containing artificial sweeteners are of no use to you in this situation. Make sure that you always carry some sort of readily available carbohydrate food. This is especially important if you are a driver or are about to exercise vigorously. For more on this, see the sections on diet (pp.19–28) and exercise (pp.54–55).

SEVERE ATTACKS

Although rare, your blood glucose level sometimes drops so rapidly that you do not have time to take the corrective action described above. You may become drowsy or unconscious and might even have a seizure. This situation is obviously frightening for both you and those around you. Take precautions to make sure that it does not happen again. Get advice from your doctor to resolve the problem. There are various ways of dealing with a person having a severe hypoglycemic attack:

● When you are not in a state to eat or drink anything, a sugary gel, which can be purchased at a pharmacy, can be squirted into your mouth or rubbed on your gums. This should not be done, however, if you are having a seizure.

● The hormone glucagon, which causes blood glucose to rise, can be injected into your arm or buttock to revive you. Then you can have something to eat or drink.

LOSING CONSCIOUSNESS
If the blood glucose level drops too rapidly, a person may become unconscious. If this happens, a sugary gel can be smeared inside the mouth or a glucagon injection given.

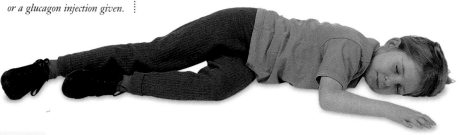

HYPOGLYCEMIA AT NIGHT

You and your family may worry about a hypoglycemic attack during sleep or the possibility of having one and not waking up. This is an especially frightening prospect when the patient is a young child with insulin-dependent diabetes mellitus (for more on this, see pp.63–67).

In reality, the problem is not that dramatic. First, you are likely to wake up due to the symptoms of a falling blood glucose level. You may feel sweaty, restless, or irritable. Your restlessness may wake your partner even if you remain asleep. It is not unusual to sleep through a severe hypoglycemic reaction. In response to the falling level of glucose, your body mobilizes various hormones that will stimulate the release of stored glucose to correct the problem. After a reaction like this, you wake up with a headache and symptoms much like a bad hangover. Sometimes, there may be a swing too far in the opposite direction, and your blood glucose rises too much. If you regularly wake up with these symptoms, take a few early morning (2–4 a.m.) blood glucose tests to see if you are having hypoglycemic reactions that you are unaware of at the time. Then you will know why you are not feeling well. Talk to your doctor about whether your nighttime dose of insulin needs adjusting or if the insulin should be changed to a different type.

HYPOGLYCEMIA IN BED
If you experience an attack while you are sleeping, the effects of falling blood glucose will probably wake you up.

HYPOGLYCEMIC AWARENESS

You may have read stories about people with diabetes complaining about losing their "early warning system" of an impending hypoglycemic reaction. People who have had diabetes for a very long time become less able to predict when they are about to have a hypoglycemic attack. The warning signs seem to become less noticeable after about 15–20 years on insulin. No one knows why this occurs. However, the ability of the pancreas to release glucagon in response to low blood glucose diminishes over time. Some people say their symptoms change. For others, symptoms come on so much faster that there is no time to take preventive action.

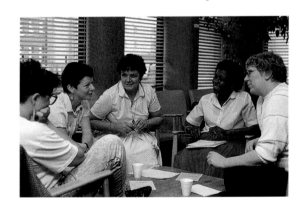

The problem is more common in people whose average blood glucose levels are on the low side of normal. Adjusting the treatment to allow the blood glucose level to rise slightly may result in the return of an old pattern of symptoms. However, any change of this kind must be discussed carefully with the diabetes care team.

DIABETES CARE TEAM
If you are experiencing frequent hypoglycemic attacks, your diabetes care team may recommend adjusting your treatment. Make sure that you meet regularly with them for advice.

MAINTAINING A BALANCE

Can hypoglycemia be avoided by constant high blood glucose levels? Yes, persistently high blood glucose levels help you avoid hypoglycemia. However, this also dramatically increases the risk of developing complications of diabetes (see pp.68–80).

Patients on insulin may find it very difficult to maintain the delicate balance between risky hyper-glycemia and troublesome hypoglycemia. However, the balance is much easier these days with the various preparations and injection devices available.

If you are having troublesome attacks followed by high blood glucose levels, consult your doctor or diabetes care team. Your treatment may need to be adjusted or changed.

KEY POINTS

- Hypoglycemia can occur in any patient taking insulin or sulfonylureas.
- Patients differ in their warning signs of hypoglycemia.
- If you think an attack may be coming on, try to confirm hypoglycemia with a blood test.
- If this is not possible, consume a fast-acting carbohydrate such as orange juice (not low-calorie).
- Milk and cookies are not ideal because they are not rapidly absorbed.
- If hypoglycemia is a recurrent problem, seek advice from your doctor or diabetes care team.

Breaking your routine

When a person who does not have diabetes exercises, the release of insulin from the pancreas stops while other hormones are produced that cause the blood glucose level to rise.

When you are being treated with insulin or sulfonylureas, your insulin level rises when you exercise. If you were to inject insulin into one of the limbs that you exercise, you might notice that the insulin is absorbed faster than usual. Therefore, it is important to let your exercise partner know that you are on insulin and tell him or her what to do if you have a hypoglycemic reaction.

EXERCISING

When you exercise, adjust your medication and/or your diet to make allowances for the impact on insulin and blood glucose. Your dose of insulin may have to be cut by as much as one-half, depending on how vigorous an exercise session you plan. Making the appropriate adjustments in your insulin dose is more difficult when you exercise unexpectedly, which is a particular problem with children. Once again, the solution is to have available a quick-acting carbohydrate snack, such as a drink, candy, or a chocolate bar.

THINKING AHEAD
If you are planning any form of vigorous exercise, you should reduce your insulin dose beforehand.

As long as you take sensible precautions, there is no reason why you should not participate fully in sports. People with diabetes can take part in just about every known sport. However, there are some, such as scuba diving or hang gliding, that require special considerations and therefore are best avoided. High-risk sports often have special rules and regulations pertaining to people with diabetes. It is particularly important for your own safety that you abide by them.

SOCIALIZING

With a little thought and planning, you can go to any party and enjoy yourself as much as ever. The main considerations about a party are that you will probably be eating later than usual, having different kinds of food, and possibly dancing late into the night. If you are on insulin, make adjustments to account for these factors. If a meal will be several hours later than normal, eat a light snack before you go and delay your injection until the meal is ready. If the party starts really late, you will probably need extra carbohydrates with your meal and your normal insulin dose. Take some extra food and perhaps a high-energy drink if you plan to keep going into the late hours.

The best plan for those who are on two daily doses of medium-acting insulin, known as a basal-bolus regimen, is to substitute a smaller dose of quick-acting insulin, plus a snack at about midnight,

Some Simple Tips for Enjoying a Night Out

There is no need for people with diabetes to avoid social occasions and parties. Follow the commonsense rules below.

- When you are on medication, eat more to allow for extra activities such as dancing.
- Never drink alcohol on an empty stomach; always have some carbohydrates first.
- Keep some quick-acting carbohydrate foods with you on a crowded dance floor in case of hypoglycemia. It may not be possible to get to a bar or dining area quickly enough.

for the overnight medium-acting insulin. A blood test about three or four hours later is a good idea. If you will be dancing, you will need additional carbohydrates. How much depends on how much energy you use.

TRAVELING

There is no reason why your diabetes should interfere with or restrict your travel plans. However, if you are going abroad, you would be wise to take out comprehensive travel insurance or make sure that your health plan covers you outside of the country.

There may be special considerations when you are going somewhere extremely remote or inaccessible. Discuss your plans with your doctor. Wherever you go, especially if it is off the beaten track, make sure that you will be able to obtain insulin or medication there if necessary, just in case you somehow lose your supplies. Never pack all your insulin in one suitcase.

You should check the immunization requirements for your destination well in advance of traveling. In some cases, several weeks are needed to complete the course of immunizations. Preventive measures of this kind may be particularly important for travelers with diabetes. It is reassuring to know that taking antimalarial drugs will not interfere with treatment for diabetes.

CROSSING TIME ZONES

If you are going on a long flight you need to plan carefully and ask your doctor for help. Remember that traveling west extends your day, and traveling east shortens it.

● **If you are on insulin** You will have fewer problems if you are on a multiple basal-bolus regimen using an injection pen than if you normally inject twice a day. For an extended day, the simplest solution is to have an extra injection of quick-acting insulin before the extra meal that will very likely be given during the flight. When you reach your destination, have your normal evening dose of insulin followed by your evening meal. The next morning, have your insulin before breakfast as usual, then try to match your eating pattern to that of the locals. However, this is not always easy if you have jet lag.

The night will probably be shorter when you are traveling east. Use a smaller dose of medium-acting insulin, perhaps 10–20 percent less than usual. Use the smaller dose either before your evening meal if you are on twice-daily injections or before you go to sleep if you are on multiple injections, followed by your usual prebreakfast dose on the next day.

You should not feel that you have to eat all the meals that are offered on the flight if you do not want or need them. Let the airline staff know that you have diabetes. Make sure that either the staff or your traveling companions know what to do if you have a hypoglycemic reaction and know how to give you insulin. Similar principles will apply if you are traveling across time zones by sea.

You do not need to have a refrigerator to store your insulin as long as you can keep it relatively cool. If this is a problem, you can use either a cold pack or a thermos.

● **When you are on medication** You should not need to make any changes to your treatment schedule. However, get the advice of your doctor before taking a very long flight.

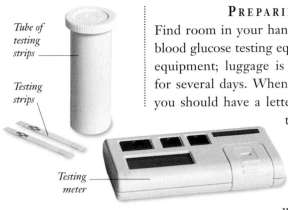

Tube of testing strips

Testing strips

Testing meter

TESTING EQUIPMENT
Make sure that you carry your blood glucose testing equipment in your hand luggage, just in case your main baggage is lost.

PREPARING FOR A TRIP

Find room in your hand luggage for your medication, blood glucose testing equipment, and any other medical equipment; luggage is sometimes lost or goes astray for several days. When carrying syringes and needles, you should have a letter from your doctor explaining that you have diabetes and how it is treated. This is especially important if you are going to certain countries in the Middle or Far East. People with diabetes should carry some form of identification card or bracelet indicating their condition and medication. The American Diabetes Association can supply cards in several different languages that identify your condition. You may never need to show either document, but it is best to have them just in case.

It is safe to take travel sickness remedies along with your diabetes treatment if necessary, but, if you know you are prone to travel sickness, take a supply of fruit juice or another sweet drink in case you cannot eat much.

In other respects, you only need to follow the same commonsense rules as any other traveler. Do not get too much sun, check the alcohol content of unfamiliar local drinks, and avoid unsanitary restaurants or street vendors.

WHEN YOU ARE ILL

Everyone gets colds and flu, which, like other illnesses, can affect the control of diabetes. The most likely result is a rise in your blood glucose level. Make frequent checks to test whether this is happening, especially if you are on insulin.

TYPE 1 DIABETES (IDDM)

Many people with type 1, or insulin-dependent, diabetes think that, if they are not eating, they should not take their insulin and that doing so would cause a hypoglycemic attack. In fact, the opposite is the case. Your blood glucose level is much more likely to be too high than too low in these circumstances. Even if you have a stomach virus and vomit constantly, you will still need some insulin to keep your glucose under control. If you cannot keep any fluids down, call your doctor immediately. Hospitalization may be necessary until you are able to eat and drink again.

TYPE 2 DIABETES (NIDDM)

If you have type 2, or non-insulin-dependent, diabetes, continuing to take your medication when you are not able to eat or drink may cause a hypoglycemic reaction. You may need a lower dose while you are ill. However, unless you are monitoring your blood glucose level regularly, you may need your doctor's advice on how to make the adjustment. If your illness does not clear up quickly, you may need to be hospitalized for a few days.

HAVING A BABY

Having diabetes is no reason to avoid having a baby. The condition does not affect fertility. You should have no problems conceiving unless you are one of the minority of women who have severe complications or whose diabetes is poorly controlled.

If you are planning to conceive in the near future, see your physician before you do. Make sure that your blood glucose levels are as well controlled as possible. In addition, folic acid supplements are highly recommended.

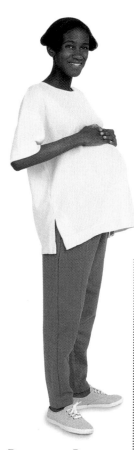

DIABETES AND PREGNANCY
Careful, regular monitoring of blood sugar levels is important before and during pregnancy. High blood glucose levels can cause the baby to grow too quickly.

Talk to your diabetes care team about your pregnancy. Special prepregnancy counseling may be available. Watch your blood glucose levels carefully when you are pregnant. High blood glucose levels, particularly in very early pregnancy, can affect a baby's development. The baby may grow too quickly or too much fluid may accumulate inside the membranes surrounding it.

Your doctor may want to see you every few weeks and recommend that you check your blood glucose more often than usual. Your insulin dose will probably double or even triple during this time, but it will return to normal after the birth. The insulin you take cannot do your baby any harm and does not lower the baby's blood glucose. There is also no need to worry that you could injure the baby by injecting into your abdomen. Hypoglycemia in the mother is not known to harm the baby in any way.

There is a good chance that you will be able to have a normal delivery. However, some women require cesarean section because their babies grow too large for normal vaginal delivery due to the diabetic mother's glucose levels being higher than normal. Your obstetric and diabetes care teams will discuss the delivery options with you beforehand. If a normal delivery is chosen, you may need a drip infusion containing insulin and a sugar solution into a vein to control your diabetes during labor.

With the advances made in recent years in the prenatal care of women with diabetes, you can look forward to a healthy pregnancy and a normal, healthy baby.

GESTATIONAL DIABETES

Some women develop diabetes for the first time when they are pregnant, after which their blood glucose levels return to normal. Usually, gestational diabetes, as it is known, can be kept under control by eating the right kinds of foods. Some women may need insulin injections. You will not be treated with oral drugs for diabetes while you are pregnant. After the birth, watch your weight and stick to a healthy diet because you now have a greater-than-normal risk of developing non-insulin-dependent diabetes later in life.

Pregnant women on insulin need to follow all the recommendations on diet, exercise, and the other issues for insulin-dependent diabetes patients as outlined in earlier chapters.

KEY POINTS

- When exercising, remember to eat extra carbohydrates or reduce your insulin or sulfonylurea medication beforehand.
- When exercising with others, tell them about your diabetes and explain what to do in the event of a hypoglycemic attack.
- At parties, never drink alcohol on an empty stomach. Always have some quick-acting carbohydrate foods available.
- If eating later than usual or having extra food, you may need to adjust your insulin.
- Review health insurance policies before any foreign travel.
- If traveling between continents, have an extra dose of insulin with your extra meal going west, and omit a scheduled meal and insulin dose going east.
- Always pack your insulin in your hand luggage.
- Carry identification indicating your diagnosis and medication regimen.
- Even if you are ill and not eating, you still need your insulin or medication.
- If you cannot take your medication or insulin because of vomiting, seek medical help.
- Diabetic women should seek early obstetric and medical advice before they become pregnant.

Children with diabetes

*T*ype 1, or insulin-dependent, diabetes usually
develops between the ages of 11 and 13. It
is unusual in children under five, although
there have been cases of babies developing
insulin-dependent diabetes within
a few days of birth.

Children are active and burn up energy,
which can make it difficult to keep their food
intake and insulin in the correct balance. Usually the
best approach is to give two or three injections a day
with each one containing some short-acting and some
medium-acting insulin.

Understandably, you will worry about your child
having hypoglycemic reactions and may therefore find
it difficult to let him or her out of your sight. However,
as a child gets older, you will probably find it easier to
allow your child the independence he or she needs
to mature emotionally.

Children can learn to inject themselves at any
age. However, you will probably want to check the
insulin doses. Injector pens have been a big help with
this problem because of their convenience and the ease
of dialing the correct insulin dose.

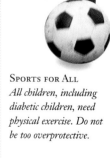

SPORTS FOR ALL
*All children, including
diabetic children, need
physical exercise. Do not
be too overprotective.*

HOME MONITORING

Blood tests can be unpleasant for young children and difficult to perform because their fingers are so small. Urine tests are often recommended instead, either alone or combined with occasional blood tests. Once your child is a bit older, you will have to encourage him or her to be conscientious about monitoring blood glucose levels on a regular basis. However, do not be surprised if he or she is resistant to it. Rebellion is a natural part of growing up. Many teenagers go through a period of refusing to cooperate with this aspect of their diabetes care. This is a difficult situation, but avoid direct confrontation as much as possible. Remember, it is much more important for your child to take insulin regularly than to perform repeated blood glucose tests.

HYPOGLYCEMIA

Children's blood glucose levels can fall quickly, especially if they are active. It may be difficult to spot the warning signs in time. Very young children may not recognize the warning signs at all. When the blood glucose level drops so low that the child becomes drowsy or unconscious, the best treatment is glucagon. Keep a supply readily available if you have a young child with diabetes. Once this treatment

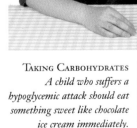

TAKING CARBOHYDRATES
A child who suffers a hypoglycemic attack should eat something sweet like chocolate ice cream immediately.

has taken effect, the child needs to have some carbo-hydrates in the form of food or a sweet drink.

Hypoglycemia is most likely to arise when the child is exercising. Therefore, the play-group leader, teacher, or whoever is responsible for the child must know exactly what to do if he or she experiences a hypoglycemic reaction. This is especially important at school. Also, make sure that the kitchen staff at school is aware of the situation to be sure that the child makes the appropriate food choices.

PROBLEMS WITH FOOD

The amount a child eats can vary by as much as 50 percent from one day to the next. Some days it is difficult to persuade children to eat anything, while at other times you cannot stop them from eating constantly. This makes life difficult if you have a child with diabetes. As a rule, give your child something to eat whenever he or she is hungry, even if this means eating more than the diet allows. As children get older, they need higher doses of insulin. Positive urine tests or high blood glucose values indicate that they need more insulin rather than less food. Low blood glucose, on the other hand, can indicate that a child needs either less insulin or more food. Discuss this with his or her diabetescare team.

BREAKING THE RULES
Children do not understand the importance of keeping to a diet, and will often drink or eat something forbidden.

Many children break the rules and secretly eat candy or chocolate. Do not cut down on their normal food intake to compensate for these extra carbohydrates. If your child is old enough to understand, try to explain calmly why cheating in this way will result in high blood glucose and may lead to complications (see pp.68–80). Discuss the situation in a calm and measured way and give your child plenty of time to ask questions.

Children with diabetes need to take the same kind of precautions as adults when their normal routine is disrupted by travel or illness (see pp.56–59). They must also learn to take care of themselves when exercising and to follow the commonsense rules outlined on pages 54–55. If you are in doubt about how to handle these situations, speak with your child's doctor.

FAMILY REACTIONS

Siblings may be jealous of the amount of extra attention given to a child with diabetes. Equally, the child may resent the need to cope with diabetes when others do not have to bother. It is important that all these feelings are brought out into the open and discussed by the whole family. Talking things over at regular intervals can help clear the air and may encourage your other children to become involved in watching for signs of hypoglycemia. If they are old enough and willing, you should teach them how to treat a hypoglycemic reaction (see pp.49–50).

One area of possible family contention occurs at mealtimes. Family members, especially children, who do not have diabetes may complain about having to eat healthy foods. However, the diet recommended for people with diabetes is the same one we should all be following. Discourage your other children from eating treats such as candy and chocolate in front of a child with diabetes. Explain the problem and try to persuade the other children that a restriction of their candy intake is good for their health.

BEHAVIORAL ISSUES

Many children quickly discover that being difficult about food is a great way to upset their parents. Children with diabetes are no exception. They may realize that refusing to eat at mealtimes or having a hypoglycemic reaction is a sure way to get attention. They may also refuse to do urine or blood glucose tests or may make up the results. This type of behavior is obviously distressing and frustrating to parents and can greatly disrupt family life. However, it is not at all unusual. Do not feel guilty if you cannot handle these problems easily. Your child's diabetes care team has seen them often and can offer help and advice. Sometimes, it is a good idea to bring in an outsider, a family friend, or a specially trained counselor, who can help the child understand the effect of his or her

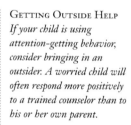

behavior. It is important to understand that this may be a child's way of expressing a deep-seated worry about his or her diabetes.

GETTING OUTSIDE HELP
If your child is using attention-getting behavior, consider bringing in an outsider. A worried child will often respond more positively to a trained counselor than to his or her own parent.

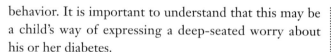

KEY POINTS

- Diabetes in children most commonly develops between the ages of 11 and 13.
- Very young children may need to rely on urine tests. Older children should be encouraged to use blood tests if possible.
- Food battles are even more common and problematic with diabetic children because of the potential risk of hypoglycemia.
- Try to avoid confrontation. If battles are upsetting the family, discuss the issues with your child's diabetes care team.

Complications of diabetes

Having diabetes does not mean that you will inevitably develop complications of the disease. Careful research has shown that the better your blood glucose control, the less likely you are to experience any problems.

The Diabetes Control and Complications Trial (DCCT), a large study of diabetes in the US, and the UKPDS study in the UK have shown that any improvement in blood glucose control will reduce your risk of developing complications. Knowing this helps many people work harder at controlling their diabetes when they are tempted to let things slide.

In addition to good diabetic control, either giving up smoking or not starting in the first place can reduce your chances of developing complications. Smoking and diabetes definitely do not mix. All of the possible complications listed in the following pages are more common in people who smoke. If you have developed any of them, it is particularly important that you stop smoking immediately. The dangers of smoking cannot be over-emphasized and may be the incentive you need to quit.

SMOKING AND DIABETES
Complications are more common in diabetic patients who smoke. Giving up cigarettes should be a priority.

High blood pressure (hypertension) also increases the risk of diabetic complications in the eyes, kidneys, and arteries. This increased risk, however, can be modified by control of blood pressure.

YOUR EYES

Diabetes can affect your eyes in various ways, ranging from temporary blurring of your vision to the more serious effects of retinopathy, damage to the light-sensitive layer at the back of the eye.

BLURRY VISION

When you first start using insulin or medication, your vision may seem a bit blurry. This is caused by dehydration of the lenses in the eyes as your diabetes develops. By rapidly lowering your blood glucose level, treatment causes a fluid shift in your eyes and may cause blurring.

Fortunately, the problem is only temporary and should clear up in a few months without the need for treatment. If you happen to need glasses, wait until the blurring has disappeared before getting a new prescription. The result of your vision test may change once your diabetes stabilizes.

CATARACTS

When you have had diabetes for a long time, you are more susceptible to cataracts because of a buildup of sugars in the lens of the eye. The sugars make the lens of the eye opaque, interfering with the transmission of light to the back of the eye, and this can be particularly annoying in bright sunlight.

Fortunately, this problem can be treated with a simple operation to replace your damaged lens with a plastic one.

Body Parts Affected by Complications

- Eyes (blood vessels supplying the retina)
- Kidneys
- Peripheral nerves in the arms, hands, legs, and feet
- Skin
- Large blood vessels

The operation can often be done under local anesthesia on an outpatient basis and is generally very successful.

RETINOPATHY

All types of diabetes can affect a highly specialized structure at the back of your eye called the retina. The central part, called the macula, enables you to see colors and fine detail. The peripheral part picks up black and white and enables you to see in the dark.

The small blood vessels supplying the retina are affected by diabetes. Small blisters or microaneurysms can form and may burst, resulting in tiny hemorrhages. Blood vessels may also leak, allowing fluid to collect on the surface of the retina, which then forms what are called hard exudates. This leakiness is usually a sign that the blood supply to that part of the eye is inadequate. When retinopathy reaches an advanced stage, new blood vessels can grow as the body tries to improve the blood supply. These new vessels are fragile and may break and bleed extensively. This condition, which is known as a vitreous hemorrhage, can seriously affect the sight.

- **Treating Retinopathy** Fortunately, laser treatment developed in recent years can greatly retard the damage caused by diabetic retinopathy. The earlier the treatment is given, the more successful it is. For this reason, have your eyes checked at least once a year. Eye exams should be performed by an ophthalmologist who is skilled in this type of examination. A few people may develop a more serious form of retinopathy called maculopathy, especially later in life. This means that the blood supply to the central part of the eye is reduced, which can seriously affect the person's ability to perceive color and fine detail. Unfortunately, laser treatment is not as successful in treating this particular problem. Nonetheless, early detection and treatment is proven to protect and preserve vision.

If you need laser treatment for retinopathy, you will be treated by a specialist. First, drops are placed in the eye to dilate the pupil, making the retina easier to see. You then put your head in a headrest to keep it still

The Structure of the Eye

The eyeball's surface has three layers: the tough outer sclera or white of the eye; the choroid, composed of blood vessels; and the retina, containing light-sensitive cells and blood vessels.

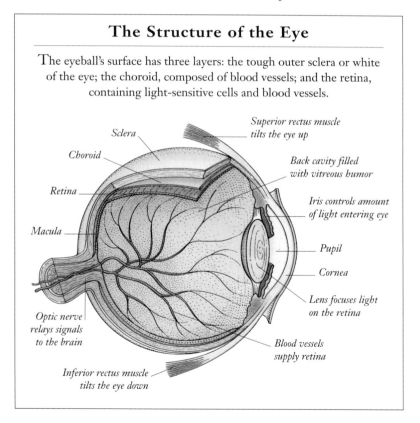

Sclera

Choroid

Retina

Macula

Optic nerve relays signals to the brain

Inferior rectus muscle tilts the eye down

Superior rectus muscle tilts the eye up

Back cavity filled with vitreous humor

Iris controls amount of light entering eye

Pupil

Cornea

Lens focuses light on the retina

Blood vessels supply retina

while the doctor uses a special camera to examine the eye and identify which parts of the retina need treatment. The treatment is usually painless. You will see brief flashes of bright light, sometimes several hundred in each treatment session, as the laser is used. You may need several sessions for each eye. Your vision may be blurry for 24–48 hours after each session.

YOUR KIDNEYS

The kidneys work as large blood filters. One of their tasks is to get rid of excess water and the by-products of everyday living. Diabetes can damage these filters because glucose accumulates in tiny blood vessels of the kidney. The effect is similar to enlarging the holes in a mesh cloth. This damage allows substances that would normally be retained to pass into your urine.

One of the substances that appears in the urine when the filters are damaged is protein. A particular protein called albumin appears at a very early stage of diabetic kidney damage. The presence of albumin in the urine is called albuminuria, and current tests can detect the presence of very small amounts, or microalbuminuria.

The availability of these tests is one reason why you are asked to provide a urine sample when you have an appointment with your doctor, even if you normally perform blood tests for glucose. Sometimes you may get a positive result from the albumin test, which is in fact caused by a urinary infection. Your urine sample is checked for this possibility.

Your doctor will want to monitor you closely if albumin is detected in your urine because of the possibility of more serious kidney damage and even kidney failure in the long term.

Monitoring kidney damage is even more important if, like many people with albuminuria, you also have high blood pressure. The two tend to go together because the kidneys also have a role in controlling blood pressure. Recent research has shown that treating high blood pressure in people with diabetes can dramatically slow the effect of diabetes on their kidneys.

At the moment, those people who do eventually suffer from kidney failure may need treatment either by dialysis, also known as a kidney machine, or by a transplant. Research is ongoing in an effort to prevent this form of kidney failure.

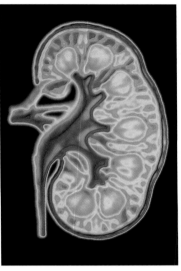

YOUR NERVES

Diabetes can affect the nerves in two ways. As with the eyes and kidneys, blood supply to the nerves may be affected. Direct damage to the nerves as a result of high blood glucose can also occur.

Nerve damage is known as neuropathy. The consequences of neuropathy depend on which of the three types of nerve is affected.

THE KIDNEY
This image shows the internal structure of the kidney. Any sign of a protein called albumin in your urine may indicate kidney damage and requires further investigation.

• **Motor nerves** These nerves carry messages to the muscles from the brain, stimulating muscle contraction. Damage to this type of nerve is known as motor neuropathy and can lead to a loss of muscle activity in the feet or hands. As a result, the toes can become clawed, and the fingers become weak. For more on the effects of diabetes on the feet, see pages 76–79.

• **Sensory nerves** These nerves detect pain, touch, heat, and other sensations and send messages back to the brain. Sensory neuropathy can make the feet very

Three Divisions of the Peripheral Nervous System

High levels of blood glucose can cause damage to each of the three types of nerve. Autonomic nerves carry instructions from the brain and the spinal cord to the glands and organs. Motor nerves carry instructions to the voluntary muscles. Sensory nerves relay body sensations to the brain from the skin and internal organs.

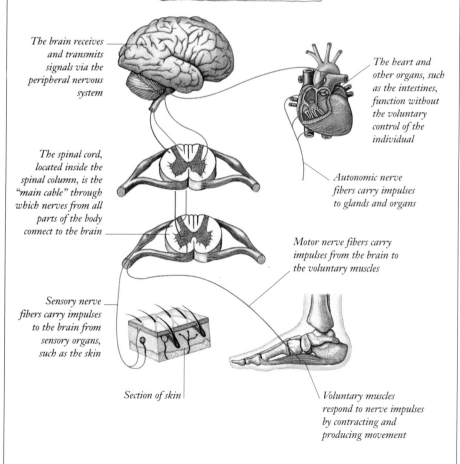

The brain receives and transmits signals via the peripheral nervous system

The heart and other organs, such as the intestines, function without the voluntary control of the individual

The spinal cord, located inside the spinal column, is the "main cable" through which nerves from all parts of the body connect to the brain

Autonomic nerve fibers carry impulses to glands and organs

Motor nerve fibers carry impulses from the brain to the voluntary muscles

Sensory nerve fibers carry impulses to the brain from sensory organs, such as the skin

Section of skin

Voluntary muscles respond to nerve impulses by contracting and producing movement sensitive and even painful at first. However, the feet eventually become numb and unable to feel any kind of sensation, including pain.

● **Autonomic nerves** These nerves are responsible for controlling automatic bodily functions such as bowel and bladder activity. Autonomic neuropathy is relatively uncommon, and its most troublesome effect is on the bladder and bowels. It can result in constipation or diarrhea that comes and goes. Occasionally, a person may suffer from persistent vomiting. Men may also be affected by a decrease in sexual potency. Most of these problems can be improved by drug treatment.

ERECTILE DYSFUNCTION

A man's ability to have a normal erection depends upon a good supply of blood through the arteries to the penis and on an intact nerve supply to constrict the veins leading from the penis. Diabetes can affect both the blood supply to the penis and the nervous control needed to constrict the veins and maintain an erection.

It is important to remember that erectile dysfunction can have psychological as well as physical causes. Whether you have diabetes or not, discuss sexual problems openly and frankly with your medical advisors. Treatment is available for all forms of erectile dysfunction.

YOUR SKIN

A small minority of people with diabetes may have skin problems caused by damage to the small blood vessels. When this occurs, reddening and thinning of the skin over the lower shin bones, a condition known as necrobiosis lipoidica, develops. Unfortunately, no effective treatment currently exists.

YOUR ARTERIES

Hardening of the arteries, which can result in heart attacks and strokes, is common in the general population. Diabetes increases your risk of developing these problems as well as of circulatory problems in the feet. Smoking and obesity also contribute to this risk, and the value to your health of smoking cessation and appropriate diet cannot be overemphasized. Problems with elevated cholesterol are common. High blood pressure (hypertension) will also increase these risks.

The management of your diabetes should include a comprehensive program for the management of all your risk factors for hardening of the arteries, both to prevent these complications and to intervene when they occur. There are now safe and effective treatments that reduce blood cholesterol levels and decrease the risk of heart attack and stroke. Particularly aggressive treatment of high blood pressure has also been shown to reduce the risk of heart attack, stroke, eye disease, and kidney disease. In addition, advances in technology have dramatically improved the available interventions for people with established problems.

YOUR FEET

You need to be aware of changes to your feet that can arise because of your diabetes and of what you can do to minimize the risk of damage. Most people with diabetes do not get serious foot problems, but even those who do can prevent things from getting worse by caring for their feet properly. Healthy circulation to your feet will help keep the tissues strong. Good circulation is aided by eating the right kinds of foods, keeping good control of your diabetes, and not smoking. Make sure that your shoes fit well and can be fastened to keep them in place without rubbing. In addition, there are specific things you can do to care for your feet. These are designed to guard against four changes that can be caused by diabetes.

● **Poor blood supply** When your circulation is restricted due to narrowed blood vessels, your feet are less able to deal with hazards such as cold weather, infection, or injury and are more susceptible to the other three changes listed below. Keep your feet warm with good-quality socks and pantyhose but avoid overheating. Be careful of seams in your socks that can press and rub, causing blisters. You should wear your socks inside out if the seams are prominent.

● **Neuropathy** Damage to the nerves makes the feet less sensitive to pain and temperature. In its early stages, people often complain of pins and needles or a feeling that they are "walking on pebbles."

When the ability of the feet to feel is reduced, a person is less likely to notice accidental injuries or infection that can lead to increased damage if untreated. In some cases, skin breaks down over a part of the foot that has experienced sustained pressure because the discomfort is not felt and the pressure is not relieved.

If you have some degree of neuropathy, you must get into the habit of checking your feet every day for any cuts or wounds. The easiest way is to make a regular foot-care program part of your daily routine. Also, check the temperature of bathwater with your hand before you get in, and avoid "toasting your toes" in front of the fire.

● **Dryness** Loss of elasticity or moisture in the skin of your feet can be associated with neuropathy

HEALTHY FEET
A daily routine is essential to keep your feet healthy and will also alert you to any changes that occur.

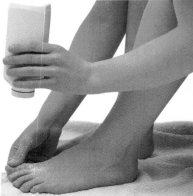

and a poor blood supply. However, dryness can develop even when you have good circulation and normal feeling.

Dry and flaky skin is much less supple due to a lack of protection by sweat and natural oils from the everyday pressures and frictions of walking.

When the skin on your feet is very dry, you are more prone to the formation of calluses and corns and to splits around the edges known as fissures. You can help replace some of the lost natural moisture by applying a good cream every day and using a foot file or pumice stone to remove dead skin. Be gentle and never use chemicals designed to remove corns and calluses or try to cut them away with blades because you could easily injure yourself.

● **Changes in the shape of your feet** These changes can take place over a period of time as a result of diabetes. The bones underneath may become more prominent due to changes in the fatty pad under the ball of your foot. The front part of your foot may spread and your toes may claw. When the tissues under your foot are strained, pain in the heel may result. Usually, these changes are a result of minor alterations in the shape of your foot. You may need new shoes to get a better fit.

EXPERT CARE

As a person with diabetes, you need to take excellent care of your feet. Many people are perfectly able to look after their own feet. However, if you have a physical or visual disability that might limit your ability to do this effectively, or if you have any of the complications listed above, you should have regular appointments with a health professional such as a podiatrist.

Caring for Your Feet

Good foot care is very important in preventing complications in diabetes and should form part of your hygiene routine. Feet should be washed and inspected daily for signs of disease.

- Wash your feet daily in warm water using a mild soap. Do not soak feet for a long time because it removes more of the precious oils from your skin. Be careful to avoid the development of soggy areas between your toes that can split or increase the likelihood of soft corns.

- Dry feet should be treated with a moisturizing cream to avoid cracks or fissures.

- Apply rubbing alcohol to white, damp areas between your toes unless there has been any bleeding. In the event of bleeding, see your doctor. Athlete's foot can be treated with rubbing alcohol or an antifungal powder or spray from the pharmacy. If it persists, see your doctor.

- Your toenails should be cut or filed straight across unless your doctor advises otherwise. Sharp corners can be smoothed with a foot file or an emery board.

- Corns and calluses are best removed by a health professional. Pads or cushion soles may be useful temporary protection for affected areas if you cannot receive medical attention immediately.

- Get medical advice immediately if you see any signs of ulceration developing anywhere on your feet.

WHAT YOU CAN DO

You may feel alarmed after reading about all these possible complications. However, they can all be prevented with careful attention to diabetes care and blood glucose control. Remember that complications are not inevitable and that you have an important role in their prevention.

KEY POINTS

- Diabetes can affect the eyes by causing cataracts or damage to the back of the eyes, a condition called retinopathy.
- Early detection and treatment of eye problems are very effective at preventing progression and loss of eyesight.
- Kidney damage occurs in a minority of patients and can be detected early by a urine test for albumin.
- Peripheral nerves can also be damaged, and feet and hands need to be checked regularly.
- Treatment is most effective when complications are detected early. Visit your doctor for regular checkups.

Diabetes care

The following medical procedures and information are what you should expect as a person with diabetes from your health-care professionals.

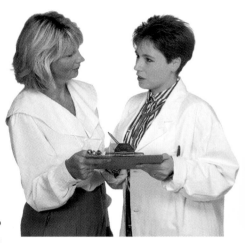

WHAT TO EXPECT

When you have just been diagnosed, you should have:

• A full medical examination.

• A discussion with a registered nurse who has special expertise in diabetes. He or she will be able to explain what diabetes is and talk to you about your individual treatment.

MEDICAL CAREGIVERS
All people with diabetes have a right to expect expert care from qualified medical advisors.

• A discussion with a registered dietitian, who will want to know what you are used to eating and will give you basic advice on what to eat in the future. A follow-up meeting should be arranged for more detailed advice.

• A discussion of the implications of your diabetes on your job, driving, insurance, and medication charges, and whether to inform the Department of Motor Vehicles and your insurance company if you drive.

• Information about services offered by the American Diabetes Association (ADA) and details of your local ADA group.

• Ongoing education about your diabetes and the beneficial effects of exercise and regular assessments of your control of the disorder.

You should feel free to take a close friend or relative with you to educational sessions.

TREATMENT WITH INSULIN

If you are treated with insulin, you should have:

• Frequent sessions for basic instruction on injection technique, taking care of insulin and syringes and pens, and blood glucose testing and what the results mean.

• Supplies of relevant equipment and dietary advice.

• A discussion about the possibility of hypoglycemia and how to deal with it.

TREATMENT WITH PILLS

If you are treated with pills, you should have:

• A discussion about the possibility of hypoglycemia and how to deal with it.

• Instruction on blood or urine testing and what the results mean.

• Supplies of relevant equipment and dietary advice.

TREATMENT BY DIET

If you are treated by diet alone, you should have:

• Instruction on blood or urine testing and what the results mean, and supplies of relevant equipment.

DIABETIC CONTROL

Once your diabetes has been reasonably controlled, you should have:

• Access to the diabetes team at regular intervals as instructed by your doctor. These meetings should provide time for discussion and assessing diabetes control.

• Ability to contact any member of the health-care team for specialist advice when you need it.

- More education sessions as you are ready for them.
- A formal medical review four times a year by a doctor experienced in diabetes.

AT YOUR QUARTERLY REVIEW

- Your weight should be recorded.
- Your urine should be tested for protein.
- Your blood should be tested to measure long-term control of glucose levels (hemoglobin A_{1C}).
- You should discuss control, including your home monitoring results.
- Your blood pressure should be checked.
- Your vision should be checked and the back of your eyes examined annually by an ophthalmologist. A photo may be taken of the back of your eyes.
- Your legs and feet should be examined to check your circulation and nerve supply. If necessary, you should be referred to a podiatrist.
- You should also have the opportunity to discuss with the specialist how you are coping with your diabetes at home and at work.

YOUR ROLE

You are the most important member of your care team, and it is essential that you understand your own diabetes to enable you to be in control of your condition.

You should ensure that you receive the described care from your local diabetes clinic, practice, or hospital. If these services are not available, you should:

- Contact your doctor to discuss the diabetes care available in your area.
- Contact the ADA (see Useful addresses, p. 92) or your local branch.

Future prospects for diabetic patients

Since diabetes is a common condition and seems to be increasing in incidence worldwide, there is a great deal of research into prevention, cures, and treatments of complications.

— CAN DIABETES BE PREVENTED? —

The ideal treatment would be to prevent diabetes. Our understanding of the causes of diabetes has increased dramatically over the last few decades, but there is still much to learn. In particular, we do not understand what triggers the damage to the small beta cells that produce insulin in the pancreas. The genes that predispose patients to this damage are being identified, but precisely what they control and how the damage is initiated remain unclear. Nevertheless, once these questions are answered, it may be possible that repairing these genes in patients at risk of diabetes could prevent them from developing the condition. Such research advances are, however, many years away.

For type 2, or non-insulin-dependent, diabetes, control of body weight and regular exercise are known to reduce the chances of developing the condition. Our understanding of the genes in this type of diabetes is much less complete, and full prevention seems a distant possibility.

CAN IT BE CURED?

Many patients ask if it is possible to have a transplant to cure their diabetes. For patients with type 1, or insulin-dependent, diabetes, this is an attractive prospect. If it were possible to isolate the small beta cells that make insulin and then either inject them or replace them in the patient, insulin production would be restored. There has been much research in this area over the last few decades, but a major problem remains with rejection of the transplanted cells. In addition, collecting the cells from the pancreas of donors is extremely laborious and time-consuming. There would never be enough of these cells to supply all of the patients who needed them.

New surgical treatment approaches, which involve trying to take cells either from animals or from small segments of the skin of patients with diabetes and transforming them into insulin-producing cells, are attracting a great deal of interest. Many problems remain with these ideas. However, trials could start within the next 5–10 years.

For people with type 2, or non-insulin-dependent, diabetes, the problem is more complicated because they may be making insulin but be resistant to its action. New drugs, such as the thiazolidinediones, were an attempt to improve insulin sensitivity, but the first of these, troglitazone, has had serious side effects in some patients. It is very likely, however, that newer ways of altering insulin sensitivity will be developed in the not-too-distant future.

Insulin itself has been chemically altered to change the rate at which it is absorbed from under the skin. This has led to the development of quicker-acting and longer-acting types. Some of these new "analogues" are already available by prescription. These treatments will provide greater flexibility to patients, particularly those with irregular mealtimes.

NEW TREATMENTS

We need to discover new treatments for the vast majority of patients to prevent or reduce the risk of their developing some of the more serious complications.

These treatments will concentrate on some of the basic mechanisms that cause eye, kidney, and nerve damage. As mentioned in the chapter on complications of diabetes, it seems that the exposure of these delicate structures to high glucose levels for a prolonged period of time causes chemical changes that lead to retinopathy, nephropathy, and neuropathy. Chemicals have been developed that interfere in this process in subtle ways. Perhaps long-term treatment with these medicines will prevent complications. Clinical trials are both ongoing and in the early stages of planning.

Careful control of blood pressure and cholesterol levels has also been shown to be effective in reducing complications. It is likely that newer treatments in these areas will be developed in the next few years.

It is important to remember, however, that much can be done to reduce the risks of problems from your diabetes by regular care not only from your diabetes care team but on your own part as well. Structured supervision and examination of your eyes, urine, blood pressure, feet, and cholesterol can indicate problems that can be treated before complications develop. The range of treatments and understanding of the disease has already greatly improved the outlook for patients with diabetes. This progress is likely to continue in the future.

Questions and answers

Some questions come up time and again when people find out they have diabetes. Here are the answers to some of the most common questions.

Will my driver's license be limited because I have diabetes?

Personal driver's licenses are regulated by each state but are not restricted or denied unless the person has been involved in an accident or received a ticket attributed primarily to diabetes.

A person with diabetes who tries to obtain a Commercial Driver's Licence, especially for driving a school bus, might encounter discrimination.

A Commercial Driver's License is required to drive all commerical vehicles. When driving on interstate highways, the US Department of Transportation prohibits any person treated with insulin from driving a vehicle. Intrastate driving is regulated by each state. Contact the local Department of Motor Vehicles for the regulations in your state.

Can I still enjoy a normal sex life?

Unless a man with diabetes has erectile dysfunction (see p.75), there is no reason why his sex life should be affected in any way. For a woman, having diabetes makes no difference in her fertility. However, it is worth noting that sexual intercourse is a vigorous activity and could cause your blood glucose level to drop and precipitate a hypoglycemic reaction.

Can diabetes affect my job?

It depends to some extent on what you do. If you are on insulin or sulfonylureas, the main factor to consider is what the consequences would be both for yourself and your colleagues if you suffered a hypoglycemic reaction. For this reason, you would have to think carefully about whether to take up a job that involves physical hazards, such as working at high altitude or being a member of a police force or fire department. However, if you are already employed in one of these areas when your condition is first diagnosed, you may be able to continue if your diabetes is well controlled and you rarely experience hypoglycemic reactions.

It is vitally important to tell your employer and colleagues that you have diabetes. It could be very embarrassing and possibly dangerous for you and for others if you were to have a hypoglycemic reaction and no one recognized it or knew what to do.

Will my children get diabetes?

For people with type 1, or insulin-dependent, diabetes mellitus (IDDM), there is a small but increased risk that their children will be affected. For unknown reasons, this is more likely if the father, rather than the mother, has diabetes. If both parents have diabetes, the risk is increased further. Current estimates indicate that the risk for a child with one parent with diabetes is about five percent, and, if both parents have the condition, it may be as high as 15 percent. For type 2, or non-insulin-dependent, diabetes (NIDDM), the situation is much less clear. Some families with special types of diabetes have a very high risk of inheritance. These are, however, a very small minority, and, for most patients with type 2, the risk of being affected with diabetes cannot be determined with any accuracy.

Will I go blind or have kidney failure with diabetes?

Since there is a tendency for diabetes to run in families, many patients have direct experience of relatives or acquaintances who have had severe complications of diabetes. However, serious eye and kidney problems affect only a minority of patients. In addition, the risks of developing problems can be greatly reduced with careful control of blood glucose. There are also many new treatments available for both eye and kidney complications that can prevent progression or deterioration provided the problem is detected at an early stage. This is why it is critical that diabetic patients get regular checkups.

Useful addresses

**American Diabetes
Association
National Service Center**
Online: www.diabetes.org
PO Box 25757
1660 Duke Street
Alexandria, VA 22314
Tel: (703) 549-1500
Tel: (800) ADA-DISC

**Hypoglycemia Support
Foundation**
Online: www.hypoglycemia.
org
PO Box 451778
Sunrise, FL 33345
Tel: (518) 272-7154

**Juvenile Diabetes
Foundation International**
Online: www.jdfcure.com
120 Wall Street, 19th floor
New York, NY 10005
Tel: (800) 223-1138
E-mail: info@jdcure.com

**National Institute of
Diabetes and Digestive
and Kidney Diseases
(NIDDK)**
Online: www.niddk.nih.
gov/health/diabetes/
diabetes.htm
One Information Way
Bethesda, MD 20892-3560
Tel: (301) 654-3327
Fax: (301) 907-8906

**National Diabetes
Outreach Program
Helpline**
Tel: (800) 438-5383

Notes

Notes

Notes

Index

A

acarbose 32
acromegaly 15
albumin 72–3
alcohol
  consumption 27, 55
  hypoglycemia 48–9
  pancreatic damage 15
  sulfonylureas 30–1
American Diabetes Association
  (ADA) 81, 83, 92
animal insulin 34
arteries, hardening 76
artificial sweeteners 24
autonomic neuropathy 75

B

basal-bolus regimen 55, 56–7
beta cells 84–5
biguanides 31–2
bleeding 39, 79
blood tests
  children 64
  diagnosis 16–18
  glycosylated hemoglobin
    17–18, 44
  self-administered 40–1,
    43–4, 67
blood vessels, damage 70–3,
  75–7
bowel trouble 75

C

calluses 78–9
carbohydrates 24, 48–50
cataracts 69
children
  blood tests 64
  diet 65–7
  exercise 54, 64–5

hypoglycemia 51, 63–4
  insulin 63–5
chlorpropamide 30
chromium 27
coma 46–7, 50–1
complications
  diabetes control 68
  eyes 69–72
  feet 73–5, 76–9
  kidneys 72–3
  mineral deficiency 27
  nerves 73–5, 77
  prevention 91
  sexual potency 75
  skin 77–8, 79
  smoking 68
  trial 68
corns 78–9
Coxsackie 14
cures 85–6
Cushing syndrome 15
cystitis 11

D

dehydration 10–11
Diabetes Control and
  Complications Trial 68
diagnosis 16–18
dialysis 73
diet
  see also meals
  children 65–6
  food to avoid 24–6
  recommended 19–28
  type 2 diabetes mellitus 14
dietitians 23, 81
disease 14–15
driving 81, 90

E

erectile dysfunction 75
exercise 48, 54–5, 64–5
eyes
  blurry vision 10, 69
  cataracts 69–70
  retinopathy 16, 70–2

F

fats 12, 24–5
feet 73, 75, 76–9
fertility 59
fiber 23–5
food see diet; meals
foreign countries 56–8

G

genetic factors 13, 84, 91
gestational diabetes 60–1
glimepiride 30
glipizide 30
glucagon 8–9, 46, 52
glucose
  absorption 32
  complications 72–84, 86
  control 34–6
  hypoglycemia 46–53
  illness 58
  kidney damage 72–3
  metabolism 10, 46
  monitoring 40–5
  pregnancy 59–61
glyburide 30
glycosylated hemoglobin test
  17–18, 44
glycogen 11

H

hands 73
heart attacks 76

high blood pressure 73
human insulin 34
hypoglycemia
  awareness 47–8, 52–3
  causes 46, 48–9
  children 51, 64–5
  coma 46–7, 50–1
  at night 51
  prevention 47–9
  sulfonylureas 30–1, 46
  symptoms 47
  treatment 49–50
  at work 90–1

I

IDDM *see* type 1 diabetes
  mellitus
identification products 58
illness 13–15, 58
inheritance 13, 84, 91
injections
  children 63
  glucagon 50
  insulin 32–9
  pain 38–9
  sites 37–8
  techniques 33, 36–9
insulin
  absorption rates 33–6, 85–6
  action 10–11
  "analogues" 85–6
  animal 34
  children 63–5
  deficiency 10–11
  discovery 8–9
  glucose levels 35–6
  human 34
  injections 32–9
  pregnancy 59–61
  production 8–9
  release 30–1
  resistance 10
  sensitivity 32, 85
  storage 57
  timing 34–6

traveling 56–8
  types 33–4
insulin injections 32–9
  prevention 85
insurance, automobile 81
islets of Langerhans 8–9

K

ketones 12
kidneys 42, 72–3, 91

L

laser treatment 70, 71–2
liver 10

M

maculopathy 70–1
meals
  see also diet
  children 65
  parties 55–6
  suggestions 21
  timing 20, 36, 48
  traveling 57–8
medical care
  abroad 56, 58
  ADA 81, 83, 92
  pregnancy 59–61
  tests 16–18, 44
  type 1 diabetes mellitus 17
  type 2 diabetes mellitus
    16–17
medication
  see also insulin
  acarbose 32
  altering dose 43, 48, 52–3
  biguanides 31–2
  complications 85
  measuring effectiveness 40–5
  sulfonylureas 30–1, 46–8, 54
  thiazolidinediones 32, 85
  travel abroad 59–60
  type 1 diabetes mellitus 32–9
  type 2 diabetes mellitus
    29–32

metformin 31–2
minerals 26
motor neuropathy 73
mumps 14

N

necrobiosis lipoidica 75
needles 36, 38–9
nephropathy 72–3, 86, 91
nervous system 73–5, 77
neuropathy 73–5, 77, 86
NIDDM *see* type 2 diabetes
  mellitus
night 35–6, 51

O

OHAs *see* oral hypoglycemic
  agents
oral glucose tolerance test 17
oral hypoglycemic agents
  (OHAs) 29–32

P

pain 38–9, 73, 77
pancreas 8–9, 13–15
pancreatitis 14
parties 55–6
polyuria 11
pregnancy 59–61
prevalence 12
prevention 84
protein 12, 24

R

regimens 34–6
renal threshold 424
repaglinide 31
retinopathy 16, 69–72, 91
rosiglitazone 32

S

salt 26
SBGM *see* self blood-glucose
  monitoring
secondary diabetes 14–15

seizures 50
selenium 27
self-administered urine tests
    40, 42–3
self blood-glucose monitoring
    (SBGM) 41–3, 45, 67
sensual neuropathy 79
sexual intercourse 75, 90
skin 75, 77–8
smoking 68
snacks 20–1, 55
sports 54–5
starch 21, 24–5
stress 15
strokes 76
sugar
    see also glucose
    children 65–7
    in diet 14, 24
    treating hypoglycemia 49–50
    in urine 7, 11, 42–3
sulfonylureas (SUs) 30–1, 46,
    54
symptoms 10–11

T

tests *see* blood tests; urine tests
thiazolidinediones 32, 85
thirst 10–11
thrush 10–11
transplants 73, 85
travel 56–8
treatment *see* complications;
    diet; hypoglycemia; insulin;
    medication
troglitazone 32, 85
type 1 diabetes mellitus
    (IDDM)
    cures 85
    description 9–12

diet 19–28
genetic factors 13
illness 58–9
infections 13–14
type 2 diabetes mellitus
    (NIDDM)
    cures 85
    description 9–12
    diet 19–28
    genetic factors 13
    illness 58–9
    lifestyle factors 14
    medication 29–32
    prevention 84

U

ulceration, feet 79
unconciousness *see* coma
urine 7, 10–11
urine tests 16, 18
    albumin 72–3
    self-administered 40, 42–3

V

viruses 13–14
vitamins 26
vitreous hemorrhage 70

W

weight
    controlling 22–3
    loss 10–11
    type 2 diabetes mellitus 12
work 81, 90–1

Acknowledgments

Dorling Ki

Mana
Ed

Desi
(

Indexi

T
permi
to tr
un

API
Scien